BEYOND COVID'S SHADOW

BEYOND COVID'S SHADOW

MAPPING INDIA'S ECONOMIC RESURGENCE

EDITED BY
SANJAYA BARU

RUPA

Published by
Rupa Publications India Pvt. Ltd 2021
7/16, Ansari Road, Daryaganj
New Delhi 110002

Sales centres:
Allahabad Bengaluru Chennai
Hyderabad Jaipur Kathmandu
Kolkata Mumbai

Anthology and Introduction Copyright © Sanjaya Baru 2021
Copyright for individual pieces vests with the respective authors

The views and opinions expressed in this book are
the authors' own and the facts are as reported by them
which have been verified to the extent possible,
and the publishers are not in any way liable for the same.

All rights reserved.
No part of this publication may be reproduced, transmitted,
or stored in a retrieval system, in any form or by any means,
electronic, mechanical, photocopying, recording or otherwise,
without the prior permission of the publisher.

ISBN: 978-93-90356-89-8

First impression 2021

10 9 8 7 6 5 4 3 2 1

The moral right of the authors have been asserted.

Printed at Thomson Press India Ltd., Faridabad

This book is sold subject to the condition that it shall not,
by way of trade or otherwise, be lent, resold, hired out, or otherwise
circulated, without the publisher's prior consent, in any form of
binding or cover other than that in which it is published.

CONTENTS

Introduction   vii

MANAGING GROWTH AND UNCERTAINTY

Emerging from the Pandemic's Shadow   3
C. Rangarajan and D.K. Srivastava

From a Tailspin to a Crash: What Needs to Be Done   24
Subramanian Swamy

COVID Economy and the May 2020 Package   38
Bibek Debroy

Designing a Post-COVID Recovery   52
Rajiv Kumar and Ajit Pai

Pandemic and the Dollar: Towards a Credible Indian Response   67
V. Anantha-Nageswaran

Policy Options for Post-COVID Growth   82
Arvind Virmani

The Political Economy of Uncertainty   93
Sanjaya Baru

THE FISCAL DIMENSION

Towards a New Framework for Federalism   111
Haseeb A. Drabu

Prepare for Stress and Pain   125
Omkar Goswami

Centre–State Lessons from the Coronavirus Pandemic   142
Indira Rajaraman

PANDEMIC AND THE PEOPLE

Towards a People-Centred Post-COVID Policy   159
Rama Bijapurkar

Building Safety Nets and Storm Shelters   173
Meghnad Desai

TRADE POLICY

Trade Policy and Post-COVID Growth   187
Jayanta Roy

Explaining India's Trade Performance   204
Biswajit Dhar

EMPLOYMENT AND MIGRATION

Reviving Manufacturing and Employment   223
R. Nagaraj

New Threats to Paid Employment of Women   242
A.V. Jose

Pandemic and Migrants: Missed Opportunities
and the Road Ahead   254
S. Irudaya Rajan

NEW ECONOMY

Bouncing Back: Technology and Sunrise Sectors   269
Amitabh Kant

Fixing India's 3Es   286
Manish Sabharwal

COVID Crisis: Digital Tech Remedies   297
R. Jagannathan

Glossary   309
Acknowledgements   313
Index   315

INTRODUCTION

The COVID-19 pandemic has put a spanner in the works of the global economy as a whole. Most international institutions have forecast negative rates of growth for the global economy and for most major economies over the next year. Earlier hopes for a V-shaped recovery of growth have been brought into question by more recent data on the pandemic and the impact of workplace lockdowns. The impact of both of these is, understandably, different for different countries, given the differing demographics, differences in levels of development, public health and availability of affordable healthcare, and the fiscal capacity of governments to intervene and restore momentum to their economies.

COVID-19 hit the world economy at a time when many major economies had become increasingly inward-looking, and world trade had been hit by this trend as well as by the trade war launched by the Donald Trump administration in the United States, primarily against China, but imposing collateral damage on the global economy. Growing uncertainty about global growth and world trade was accentuated by the physical disruption of the movement of people, goods and services imposed by comprehensive lockdowns in many major economies. India was no exception. In fact, India has emerged as one of the more adversely affected economies.

The Indian economy had entered an uncertain phase even before the lockdown, with several macroeconomic indicators raising concern about a loss of momentum. The annual average rate of growth of national income for India, which was around

3.5 per cent for three decades after independence (1950–80), had risen to 5.5 per cent in the last two decades of the last century (1980–2000) and had further accelerated to 7.5 per cent in the first decade of the twenty-first century. Most analysts assumed India was on a rising growth trajectory and India's potential growth rate was around 8 per cent. However, a sharp decline in the investment ratio after 2012, falling from over 35 per cent in the early 2010s to less than 30 per cent by 2019, signalled a slowdown both on account of demand and supply constraints.

While the government has tried to stimulate both demand and supply through various policy measures, the overall outlook for the economy has not been robust, with the 'animal spirits of private enterprise' considerably dampened. The new uncertainties injected by the pandemic into the minds of consumers, investors, salaried employees, workers and every segment of society have only made the situation worse, calling for a more concerted policy response. The lockdown has succeeded in accentuating the slowdown, with negative growth in the fiscal year 2020–21 likely to be followed by years of gradual recovery. Opinion is divided among analysts on the shape of the recovery curve—V, U, L, W or K—and the pace of recovery.

This volume examines the impact of the lockdown on the economy, evaluates the government's policy response and offers options for the way forward. We reached out to a diverse set of writers to offer varying and differing perspectives on the economic situation and the way forward. We invited two functionaries of the government, Rajiv Kumar and Amitabh Kant, and the chairman and a member of the Prime Minister's Economic Advisory Council (PMEAC), Bibek Debroy and V. Ananta-Nageswaran to present their views. We also invited the chairman of the PMEAC in the Manmohan Singh government, C. Rangarajan, to offer his perspective. Among the strong critics of the government who have written for this volume are the eminent economist and

Member of Parliament (MP), Subramanian Swamy and former finance minister of the erstwhile state of Jammu and Kashmir, Haseeb Drabu. We also invited several highly regarded analysts and commentators who have written extensively on various aspects of the economy to write for this volume. Each of them is respected for their intellectual integrity and professionalism. Opinions gathered here are varied and often conflicting, and offer different perspectives on the nature of the post-COVID economy.

Most authors draw attention to the fact that India's economic slowdown preceded the lockdown. C. Rangarajan and D.K. Srivastava believe that the Indian economy was already on a downslide prior to being impacted by the pandemic's economic shock in 2020–21. Even as the economy emerges from this shock, they argued, the underlying downward growth trends and factors that were driving these would still be there. Hence, considering the policy options for restoring growth momentum, they believe policy reforms are essential to overcome both the immediate challenges facing the economy as well as the underlying structural and cyclical factors that have impacted the growth momentum.

Bibek Debroy was among the first to draw attention to the problem of 'uncertainty' triggered both by the pandemic and the lockdown. He believes that the series of economic reforms introduced by the government, even before COVID struck, will hold the economy in good stead as it recovers from the impact of the pandemic and the lockdown. Endorsing his optimism, Arvind Virmani lists out 12 policy options aimed at restoring the growth momentum. Some of his proposals have already become policy. Virmani seeks a proactive industrial policy aimed at ensuring an increase in the share of manufacturing, and advises that recent restrictions on the trade and tariff policy front should be targeted only at a few countries while a free trade policy should be adopted towards the rest of the world.

Rajiv Kumar and Ajit Pai assert that the economy was on the

verge of picking up speed, thanks to policy reforms initiated since 2014, but the pandemic acted as a break, delaying what they call a 're-acceleration' of growth. They also emphasize the importance of sustained economic reforms, because the global environment has become less hospitable to emerging economies. In this context, they emphasize the need to increase investment to create efficient infrastructure, improve logistics and provide energy and capital inputs at globally comparable rates to the domestic industry, so as to improve its global competitiveness.

On an equally upbeat note, Amitabh Kant asserts that the initiatives being undertaken by the central government as part of the prime minister's (PM's) Atmanirbhar Bharat initiative will restore the economy's growth momentum. Kant lists out a series of initiatives taken by the government with the objective of making the economy more globally competitive. Sharing perspectives with Kant and Virmani, R. Jagannathan offers a menu of policy options for a post-COVID economy, emphasizing the need to create new employment opportunities in the services and digital economies. The post-COVID reform agenda is further elaborated by Manish Sabharwal, who lays emphasis on the role of investment in education, skill development and improving the productivity of labour as being key to the acceleration of growth. Sabharwal believes the COVID crisis has weakened resistance to long overdue reforms in financialization, formalization, urbanization, industrialization and skilling, and that the government should strike when the iron is hot.

The optimism on economic revival is balanced by the strikingly negative assessment of the distinguished economist, Subramanian Swamy, who presents a stinging criticism of Modi government's leadership on the economic policy front, describing it as random, unstructured and devoid of clarity on economic priorities. With no objectives set, the policy lacks a clear strategy, both for mobilizing the required resources and utilizing them in an optimal manner. An obvious example is the manner in which the target of increasing national income to $5 trillion by 2024 was set, without explaining how the required growth rate of 14.4 per cent per year would be attained. Offering a menu of policies that need to be pursued to step up economic growth, Swamy sets down two principles that must guide policy. These are: (a) incentives, rather than coercion, should be deployed to shape individual behaviour, and the government should make no promise to the people without specifying the sacrifice required to be made by them to make it happen; (b) it should be the aim of policy to make India a globally competitive economy with assured access to the markets and technological innovations of the US and some of its allies, such as Israel. Swamy suggests that the concomitant political obligations of such a strategy will have to be accepted.

Fiscal policy and the fiscal implication of post-COVID economic growth are major concerns of several of our writers. In a seminal essay on federalism, Haseeb Drabu points to how the union government's policy response across many fronts has raised questions about its commitment to the constitutional principles of fiscal federalism. He makes a powerful case for what he calls 'lateral federalism' as opposed to the current practice of 'vertical federalism'. Excessive policy centralization not only goes against the grain of fiscal federalism but imposes economic costs. Omkar Goswami surveys the fiscal landscape, drawing attention both to the challenge posed by the limitations imposed on revenues by the roll-out of the Goods and Services Tax (GST) and, more specifically, the parlous condition of state government finances. Goswami echoes Swamy's pessimism on the prospects of economic resurgence in the near future.

R. Nagaraj considers options for making the Atmanirbhar Bharat strategy work, given the various structural constraints holding back investment and growth. He believes major structural reforms can wait but what needs to be done now is to revive demand and economic momentum. Towards this end, he suggests restoring lost jobs as a priority. He also emphasizes the need for an emergency plan to double public health expenditure and the boosting of investment demand to revive economic growth aimed at reducing poverty and generating employment. A.V. Jose examines the implications of reduced employment for women in the workforce, and Irudaya Rajan surveys the challenges posed by migration and migrant labour for economic development across the country.

In the policy discussion on the response to COVID, many have pointed to Kerala's superior example. Indira Rajaraman discusses the way in which Kerala has responded to the public health challenge. Meghnad Desai offers ideas for building on some of Kerala's initiatives by strengthening safety nets and building 'storm shelters'. Desai's emphasis on building a stronger foundation for a 'welfare state' is also reflected in Rama Bijapurkar's essay on the need for a more 'people-centered' policy framework. Both draw attention to the fact that the pandemic and the lockdown have exposed structural flaws in the economy and society, impacting the poor more than the rich.

Turning to the external economy, Jayanta Roy makes a strong case for India remaining open to international trade flows, reversing the recent slide into defensive protectionism. Given Roy's intimate knowledge of Indian trade policy, his menu of policy options provided here are required to be taken seriously. Roy believes that the pre- and post-pandemic trade policy developments have weakened multilateralism in trade and that the World Trade Organization (WTO) is in a state of existential crisis. Roy advocates signing or widening trade deals with the US, European Union (EU), Japan, South Korea and the Association of Southeast Asian Nations (ASEAN), while finding ways to deal with technical barriers to trade. Warning against allowing 'atmanirbharta' (self-reliance) from turning into neo-protectionism, Roy suggests that trade policy should be formulated by a national trade policy council reporting directly to the PM.

While Roy makes a strong case for trade liberalization, Biswajit Dhar is sceptical about whether trade liberalization of the past, especially the many free trade agreements signed, have benefitted export growth. While China took advantage of India's trade liberalization in the period 2000–10, India's inability to promote the competitiveness of its own domestic industry prevented it from taking a similar lead. Dhar believes the inability of successive governments to take appropriate measures to prepare India's manufacturing sector to face the challenges of an open economy has been a key impediment in India benefitting from globalization. While India has taken several measures to deal with the trade imbalance with China—some of these measures were prompted by the border clash and the military stand-off—Dhar concludes that to facilitate post-COVID economic recovery and to promote export growth to China and the rest of the world, the government has to have a medium-term strategy for the revival of domestic manufacturing.

While the government may have some policy space on the foreign trade front, it must remain focused on the likely consequences of the economic slowdown at home and abroad for the capital account. V. Ananta-Nageswaran believes that there is a possibility that global economic instability as a consequence of the pandemic could trigger 'the end of the US dollar's reign', as he puts it, as the principal global reserve currency. Much would depend on actions that China is likely to take to consolidate its post-pandemic gains. Ananta-Nageswaran also believes that other emerging economies would have to make major policy choices of their own, given this uncertainty, and pursue their own national growth and exchange rate management strategies independent of what Western economies do. As for India, he advocates embracing sweeping structural reforms and a strong currency.

Economic policymaking is, at the best of times, an exercise based on a variety of assumptions about human response to economic incentives and disincentives. Much theorizing and policy formulation have been based on the classic assumption of *ceteris paribus*, but the pandemic has underscored the fact that 'other things are not equal'. As I conclude in my essay on the political economy of uncertainty, the defining reality of the post-COVID world is uncertainty about the behaviour of consumers, savers, investors, workers and entrepreneurs. Their confidence in the future has been shaken and shaped by a new kind of uncertainty that one normally associates with an all-out global war. Never after World War II has the entire world economy been exposed to uncertainty about the response of economic agents to policy signals. The novel coronavirus is indeed a novel experience for economic policymakers. Bringing the economy back to its medium-term trajectory of growth requires imaginative policymaking and rebuilding confidence in the narrative of India's growth story. It is not just about getting the economic policy right, but also about getting governance and national priorities right.

MANAGING GROWTH AND UNCERTAINTY

EMERGING FROM THE PANDEMIC'S SHADOW

C. Rangarajan and D.K. Srivastava

The outbreak of COVID-19 has taken the world by surprise, and its impact is now felt by almost every country. The world is experiencing an additional slowdown on top of the contracting tendencies already present, and India is no exception. The economic crisis that we are facing today is vastly different from any crisis that we have seen recently. This is the first economic crisis in recent memory that has been triggered by a non-economic factor—a pandemic. It has brought to a grinding halt nearly all economic activity.

Many multilateral bodies, financial institutions and rating agencies have recently reassessed their positions regarding India's growth prospects in 2020–21. The International Monetary Fund (IMF) has revised its forecast for 2020–21 from 1.9 per cent in April 2020 to (-)4.5 per cent in June 2020. The World Bank also revised down India's 2020–21 real gross domestic product (GDP) growth to (-)3.2 per cent from 2.2 per cent (average) over the same period. In this article, we consider India's growth prospects and policy options as the country emerges from the pandemic's shadow. The Indian economy was already on a downslide prior to being impacted by the pandemic's economic shock in 2020–21.

Note: The authors would like to thank Muralikrishna Bhardwaj, Tarrung Kapur and Ragini Trehan for their helpful inputs.

Even as the economy emerges from this shock, the underlying downward growth trends and the factors that were driving these would still be there. In considering the policy options for uplifting India's growth to reach closer to its potential, policy reforms to overcome the immediate challenges as also the underlying structural and cyclical factors besetting the growth momentum should be considered.

Economic Impact of the Pandemic

The economic impact of COVID-19 on India can be traced through four channels: (1) external demand, (2) domestic demand, (3) supply disruptions and (4) financial market disturbances.

External Demand

As the economies of the developed countries slow down and move into recession, their demand for imports of goods will go down and this will affect our exports, which even now are not doing well. In fact, after six months of negative growth, it was only in February 2020 that the Indian exports showed positive growth. Since February 2020, the growth rate has turned negative again. In April 2020, it was as high as 60 per cent (Chart 1). The pace of contraction reduced to 36.5 per cent in May 2020. The extent of decline will depend on how severely the other economies are affected. The growth rate of advanced countries is expected to be negative at (-)8 per cent.[1] Not only merchandise exports, but service exports will also suffer. Besides the IT industry, the travel, transport and hotel industries will be affected. The only redeeming feature in the external sector is the fall in global crude oil prices. India's oil import bill will come down. But this will adversely

---

[1] International Monetary Fund. (2020, June). 'A Crisis Like No Other, An Uncertain Recovery'. World Economic Outlook (WEO) Update.

Chart 1: Monthly growth (year on year) in merchandise exports

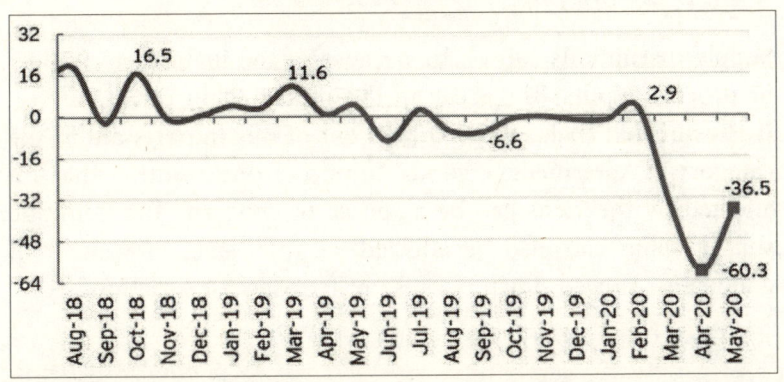

Source: Ministry of Commerce and Industry, Government of India

affect the oil-exporting countries, which absorb Indian labour. Consequently, remittances may slow down.

Domestic Demand

Domestic demand comprises three elements—private consumption expenditure, public consumption expenditure and investment. As growth slows down, private consumption expenditure will also show a declining trend. Perhaps, some sectors will be affected more severely than others. For example, as people travel less because of lockdown, the transportation industry—road, rail and air—will suffer a severe setback. Public consumption will be high because of various expenditures that the government has to undertake. Investment demand can be broken into private investment and public investment. There is an attempt to increase public investment. This aspect is discussed in detail later in the chapter. The 2019–20 corporate income tax rate reform provides additional incentive for investment in manufacturing.

However, private investment may take time to pick up.[2]

Supply Disruptions

Supply disruptions can occur because of the inability to import or procure inputs. The break in the supply chain can be severe. It is estimated that nearly 60 per cent of our imports are in the category of 'intermediate goods'. Imports from countries that are affected by the virus can be a source of concern. The domestic supply chain can also be affected, as inter-state movement of goods also slowed down because of lockdown restrictions.

Financial Market Disturbances

Financial markets respond quickly and sometimes irrationally to a pandemic like COVID-19. The entire reaction is based on fear. The stock market in India initially collapsed (Chart 2), with the indices touching a three-year low. However, they have recovered since then. It is difficult to understand the factors that move the stock market. Foreign portfolio investors initially showed great nervousness and the safe haven doctrine operated. In the process, the value of the rupee in terms of the dollar fell (Chart 3). But it has also stabilized. The revival of the stock market in India and abroad led the IMF to remark that 'the rebound in financial market sentiment appears disconnected from shifts in underlying economic prospects'.[3]

---

[2] C. Rangarajan and D.K. Srivastava. (2019, 03 October). 'The macro arithmetic of corporate tax cuts'. *Hindu Business Line*; https://www.thehindubusinessline.com/opinion/the-macro-arithmetic-of-corporate-tax-cuts/article29586882.ece
[3] Ibid.

Chart 2: Standard and Poor's Bombay Stock Exchange (BSE) Sensex Closing Value (weekly)

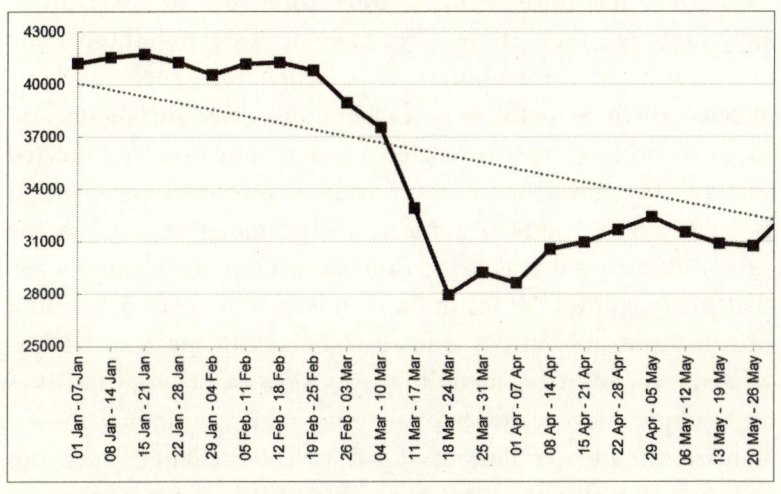

Source: BSE Official Website (bseindia.com)

Chart 3: Exchange rate movement (weekly)

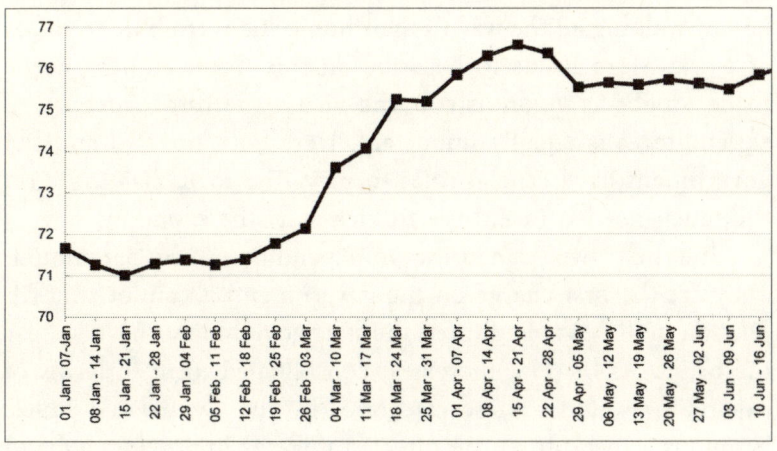

Source: Financial Benchmarks India Pvt. Ltd. (www.fbil.org.in)

Demand for Government Expenditures

COVID-19 has brought in its wake three sets of government expenditures that have become necessary. These are: (1) healthcare expenditures, (2) relief to people directly affected, such as daily wage earners and migrant labour, and (3) expenditure to stimulate demand and revive affected sectors. The government must immediately address the first two categories. There is some concern among experts on the extent of testing that is being done currently. Many experts feel that the magnitude of testing must increase manyfold. The first priority is to mobilize adequate resources to meet all health-related expenditures, including extension of hospital facilities and supply of accessories/equipment, like ventilators, masks, sanitizers and material inputs, for tests. The challenge here is not only fiscal but also organizational. The second set of expenditures tries to take care of people who have been directly affected by the lockdown. Here again, there is a feeling that the problems of those thrown out of employment have not been adequately addressed. It has been a heart-rending sight to view the migrant labour walking all the way to their home states from their places of work. More needs to be done on this front. Hunger needs to be fought as vigorously as the virus. The third category of expenditures is equally important. Here both the RBI and the government have crucial roles to play. The focus has to be on the much-needed incentives to kick-start the economy.

The first two categories of expenditures are paramount. They are the first charge on the government. It cannot stint. In relation to these expenditures, the state governments have to bear the brunt. As of now, there's no consolidated form in terms of expenditures under these categories by the Centre and states. 'Stimulus' expenditures are directed towards improving demand and offsetting disadvantages imposed on business entities to start activities. It needs to be understood that in the Keynesian sense, all increase in expenditures act as a stimulant of demand. That is how the expression 'Digging holes and filling them up' came into usage. In a broader sense, even increased expenditures in healthcare are demand-enhancing. However, analysts do make a distinction among expenditures depending on the fiscal multiplier. The expenditure under the category of 'stimulus' will be determined not only by what is needed but also what is feasible.

Monetary Policy

Monetary policy measures have come in quick succession post COVID-19. The Monetary Policy Committee (MPC) was convened once, ahead of its scheduled date. Thus, the RBI has been proactive. The various measures taken by the RBI fall under three categories: (1) policy rate changes, (2) augmenting liquidity and (3) regulatory adjustments. The policy rate under the Liquidity Adjustment Facility has been brought down to 4 per cent in May 2020 from 5.15 per cent in mid-March 2020. The magnitude of the last reduction was 40 basis points, and that of the previous one was 75 basis points. The reverse repo rate now stands at 3.35 per cent. The stance of monetary policy is accommodative. The reduction of policy rate started even before the advent of COVID-19, and gathered momentum from end-March 2020. The low reverse repo rate is expected to discourage banks from placing 'surplus' funds with the RBI. The regulatory adjustments are expected to provide relief to banks, so that their ability to expand credit may be facilitated. The numbers of refinance facilities introduced by the RBI are expected to accelerate the flow of credit to micro, small and medium enterprises (MSMEs), mutual funds and non-banking financial companies (NBFCs).

One of the important elements in the monetary policy package is to augment the liquidity in the system. This enables the banks and other financial institutions to expand credit. Another objective is to direct the liquidity in certain directions. Open market operations and augmentation of foreign exchange reserves lead to increase in durable liquidity. From end-March 2020 to early July 2020, the foreign exchange reserves of the RBI increased from $476 billion to $513 billion. This will enhance liquidity. The RBI also reduced the cash reserve ratio from 4 per cent to 3 per cent, which had the effect of increasing primary liquidity by as much as ₹1,37,000 crore. The RBI has been announcing from time to time its schedule of open market operations. It has been conducting long-term repos. In a slight modification, in March 2020, the RBI announced Targeted Long-Term Repo Operations, where it specified that the liquidity availed under this facility had to be invested in investment-grade corporate bonds and commercial paper. The RBI also extended additional refinancing facilities to the Small Industries Development Bank of India and the Export-Import Bank of India.

Regulatory changes to help the flow of credit were of several types. One important measure was the moratorium on instalments falling due for term loans. Initially, it was given for three months and later extended for another three months. Other measures include the deferment of interest on working capital facilities and the easing of working capital financing without the downgrade of asset classification. There are several more that are not listed here.

Two questions arise with respect to monetary policy measures. First, are they adequate and in the right direction? Second, what will be their effect on the overall economy? The policy rate at 4 per cent is perhaps the lowest it can get, given India's conditions. While the industry and others welcome the lowering of the rate, the savers have their own concerns. World over, there is a continuing debate as to whether savings are interest-sensitive. While there can be some doubt about the impact on overall savings, financial savings are impacted, and this is particularly so when returns on alternative assets like gold are rising. In any case, savers are already feeling the pinch. The various liquidity-enhancing measures taken together amount to our model of 'quantitative easing'. We have to note that quantitative easing took a long time to have an impact on the developed economies post 2008. While the direction of monetary policy may be right, there are two concerns. First, it is not clear whether the availability of credit is the most binding constraint on growth. More importantly, policymakers should not put too much pressure to lend. Making resources available is important and the central bank should certainly do that. It is in this sense that the measures taken so far are in the right direction. But bankers must not abdicate their responsibility to exercise judgement. They should neither be adventurous nor timid. The loans of today should not become the non-performing assets (NPAs) of tomorrow. This is certainly not an argument against lending. It is only a note of caution. Second, the central bank needs to keep a tab on the extent of the liquidity it is injecting. It is not only the private sector that is looking for liquidity but also the government. Expansion in liquidity unaccompanied by a real sector response in terms of output can lead to problems later, not necessarily in this year. It may also have to be noted that the expansion in money supply depends not only on the initial injection of liquidity by the central bank but also on subsequent credit expansion. This is elaborated in the next section on fiscal policy. It had earlier been questioned as to why monetary policy had not had any effect so far. This was when India was still in a state of lockdown. The fact was that unless the lockdown was lifted, and production started moving, banks could not lend. They may have sanctioned the loans but they would release them only when production started. Without action on withdrawing the lockdown, the economy could not move fast.

Fiscal Policy

Fiscal policy has an important role to play in the situation in which India and other countries are currently placed. However, the ability to play a big role is constrained by the fact that the fiscal position of the Government of India was difficult even before the advent of COVID-19. The fiscal deficit of the central government for 2019–20 turned out to be higher. It stood at 4.6 per cent[4]. In fact, even without COVID-19, the fiscal deficit of the centre for 2020–21 would turn out to be higher. With COVID-19, the situation gets worse. The revenue calculations of the Budget were made on the assumption that the nominal income of the country would grow at 10 per cent. With low expectations of real growth, nominal income may grow, at best, at 5 per cent[5] in 2020–21. There will thus be a deep decline in nominal growth. Analysts estimate that the tax and non-tax revenue and non-debt capital receipts in the current fiscal may fall well short of the budget estimates by a margin of close to ₹5 lakh crore. This shortfall may amount to about 2.4 per cent of GDP. The central government has already announced a revised borrowing programme for 2020–21, according to which, the estimated fiscal deficit may amount to 5.7 per cent of GDP. This deficit will have to be further increased to accommodate the additional burden arising on account of the additional stimulus package and to

---

[4]Controller General of Accounts (CGA), Government of India. (2020). 'Monthly Accounts'.

Shaktikanta Das. (2020, July 11). 'Indian Economy at a Crossroad: A view from Financial Stability Angle', Speech at the 7th SBI Banking and Economics Conclave organized by the State Bank of India; *https://www.rbi.org.in/Scripts/BS_SpeechesView.aspx?Id=1097*.

[5]This is implicit in the stimulus package announced by the finance minister in May 2020; https://pib.gov.in/PressReleasePage.aspx?PRID=1624651; https://static.pib.gov.in/WriteReadData/userfiles/Aatma%20Nirbhar%20Bharat%20%20Presentation%20Part%205%2017-5-2020.pdf

finance the National Infrastructure Pipeline (NIP). There may also be scope for some expenditure restructuring.

The series of stimulus measures announced by Finance Minister Nirmala Sitharaman are a mix of already budgeted expenditure, additional expenditure, extension of credit facility with government guarantee for certain select sectors and a host of reform measures that are indeed welcome.[6] Perhaps, it would have been useful if a more analytical distinction of expenditures had been given. Analytically, the overall stimulus package of ₹20.97 lakh crore can be divided into a budgetary and a non-budgetary part. The non-budgetary part, accounting for nearly 85 per cent of the overall package, consists mainly of liquidity-enhancing measures for banks and NBFCs, which may facilitate the financial sector in playing a key role to kick-start the economy. The credit guarantee provided by the government under the various schemes announced recently is of central importance in this context. In fact, for certain schemes, the government has come forward to provide 100 per cent guarantee, which should quicken the pace of credit sanction and delivery by banks. This will have fiscal implications only in the subsequent years. The production of goods and services is interrelated in an economic system. Once production starts, different sectors will be mutually supportive since different industries and service providers are locked in an input–output system.

The budgetary part amounts only to about 15 per cent of the overall package. This can be further divided into government expenditure that was already budgeted in the 2020–21 Budget and expenditures constituting genuine additionality. The latter component is only 10 per cent of the overall package, equivalent to nearly 1 per cent of GDP. Adding this to the enhanced level of

---

[6]C. Rangarajan and D.K. Srivastava. (2020). 'Slower growth and a tighter fiscal.' *The Hindu*; https://www.thehindu.com/opinion/lead/slower-growth-and-a-tighter-fiscal/article31538125.ece.

5.7 per cent of GDP, the Centre's fiscal deficit may be close to 7 per cent of GDP. In fact, the actual deficit may turn out to be higher.

With this high fiscal deficit, the composition of government expenditure becomes critical. Some of the establishment expenditures and subsidies, especially those linked to petroleum prices like fertilizer and petroleum subsidies, may be reduced while expenditure on health-related items may be increased. The central government has announced the freezing of increments of dearness allowance and dearness relief components in the case of salaries and pensions, respectively.

According to the NIP, the Centre's budgetary contribution to infrastructure is estimated at 1.25 per cent of GDP on an annual basis. This is less than 18 per cent of its estimated fiscal deficit in 2020–21, indicating a very poor quality of fiscal deficit. One dimension of expenditure restructuring should be to front-load infrastructure spending, including that on health infrastructure, thereby taking advantage of the higher multiplier effects associated with capital expenditures. Investment augmentation also supports demand and generates employment and income.

Support to demand will come not only from the Centre but also from the states and public sector undertakings. States have been allowed to borrow an additional 2 per cent of their respective gross state domestic product (GSDP) subject to certain conditions. In fact, at the present juncture, these conditions are not required since the enhancement of the borrowing limit is for one time, while the reforms linked to conditions are permanent in nature. In any case, states should be encouraged to support demand by going up to the full extent of the enhanced limit.

Financing of the National Infrastructure Pipeline

An important source of generating demand can be through the successful financing of the proposed NIP, which is planned from

2019–20 to 2024–25. It is meant to be financed by the central and state governments along with their public sector enterprises and the private sector. The time path of the ambitious infrastructure investment plan amounting to ₹111 lakh crore is such that it peaks in two years, namely, 2020–21 and 2022–23 (Chart 4). As Chart 5 indicates the investment peak is even more marked in the case of construction.[7] Successful financing of infrastructure in the current year and the next can be an important strategy for uplifting the economy out of the pandemic's shadow.

Chart 4: Gross fixed capital formation (GFCF) in infrastructure spending, excluding construction (₹lakh crore)

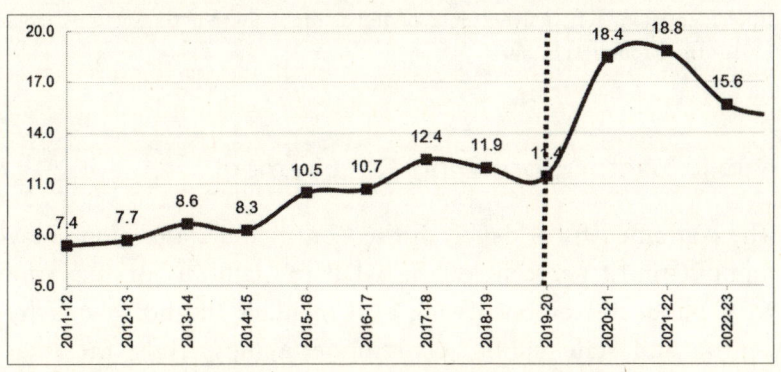

Source: National Accounts Statistics (2019), Ministry of Statistics and Programme Implementation, NIP, Government of India, Input–Output transactions table (2015–16), Brookings India

---

[7]Ernst and Young Economy Watch, various issues (2020, April, May and June); https://www.ey.com/en_in/tax/economy-watch.

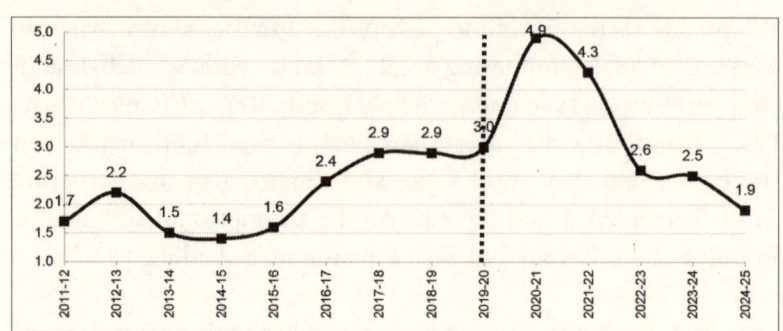

Chart 5: GFCF in construction sector (₹lakh crore)

Source: National Accounts Statistics (2019), Ministry of Statistics and Programme Implementation, NIP, Government of India, Input–Output transactions table (2015–16), Brookings India

Public Sector Borrowing Requirement

The combined fiscal deficit of the Centre and states alone may amount to 12 per cent of the GDP in 2020–21. Besides, the total public sector borrowing also includes the borrowing by central and state public sector undertakings. Thus, the total public sector borrowing requirement may well exceed the available sources of financing, consisting of the financial savings of the household sector and the savings of the public sector and net capital inflows.[8] In this context, monetizing debt has become unavoidable. The Centre must be forthcoming on these issues while recognizing that extraordinary situations call for extraordinary solutions.

---

[8] C. Rangarajan and D.K. Srivastava. (2020). 'Slower growth and a tighter fiscal.' *The Hindu*; https://www.thehindu.com/opinion/lead/slower-growth-and-a-tighter-fiscal/article31538125.ece.

How high can fiscal deficit go? The IMF, in its June 2020 update of the WEO, estimated the fiscal deficit of India and China at 12.1 per cent of GDP. All the other countries except US have a deficit lower than this. The US has a complicated procedure in determining the budget. It is not clear how far the president will succeed in pushing the expenditures. Besides, dollar as a reserve currency has its own advantages. Coming back to India's fiscal deficit, there aren't adequate resources to support a fiscal deficit of 12 per cent of GDP. Financing of the NIP may require it to be increased further. All this will require substantial support from RBI, which will have to take it on itself, either directly or indirectly, a part of the central government debt. The question ultimately relates to the extent of debt monetization that may be undertaken.

Monetization of debt can be either direct or indirect. In the indirect mode, the RBI provides liquidity to banks, which then take on a part of the debt. In the direct mode, the RBI takes on the debt directly from the government at an agreed rate. It took India long to move away from the automatic monetization of debt. It happened in the early 1990s. Even if RBI wants to support the borrowing programmes, it should not do so directly. The indirect method is preferable as the market still sends out the signals on an interest rate. In both cases, the RBI is the provider of liquidity. In fact, the government wants to borrow more at a lesser rate!

Another question pertains to whether or not the increase in primary liquidity (reverse money) automatically leads to an increase in money supply. It depends upon the money multiplier, which again depends on credit expansion by the banking system. In fact, the post-2008 phenomenon in the US and other developed countries is a good example. Despite quantitative easing, there was no price increase because lending was poor and money supply expansion was limited. This need not necessarily be the case in India. There is a strong pressure on the banks to expand credit. Therefore, the expected increase in money supply can be substantial, leading to inflation, although with a lag. This possibility cannot be ruled out. After all, many analysts forecast nil or negative increase in overall output in 2020–21. In that context, a substantial increase in money supply can lead to inflation. The only way to avoid such a situation is to ensure that credit expansion is prudent and justifiable.

Limit to Monetization of Debt

To argue as if there is no limit to monetization of debt is to ignore our own history. The critical concern is the impact of excessive liquidity on the economy. Money stock, once increased, stays. Increase in money and credit only facilitate expansion in output. If output increase slackens, increased stock of money cannot but have an impact on prices. The fear of inflation in the current year may seem unrealistic, but it can come with a lag. The high inflation post 2011 was preceded by a hefty fiscal deficit. Given the current situation of economic slack, some degree of monetization of debt is acceptable. But to assume and act as if there is no limit to monetization of debt is equivalent to storing up problems for tomorrow. Thus, the approach should be to keep government expenditures at a high level with a cautionary note on monetization of debt.

Reforms: The Next Round

Even as we take steps to kick-start the economy, we must consider the shape of the next round of reforms that would pave the way for sustained growth in the post-COVID era. However, in the case of reforms, we have reached a new stage. General reforms cutting across industries and sectors have been critical in the early stages. The earlier regime of controls and permits had to be brought to a close. But now reforms have to focus on specific sectors. Applying the general principles of liberalization to sectors such as agriculture, and particularly agricultural marketing, the power sector and telecom have assumed importance. Labour market reforms are needed across all the states. But labour reforms are introduced better when the economy is on the upswing. Consensus-building is critical before introducing labour reforms. Land markets need to be freed up, consistent with the concerns of small and marginal farmers. Financial and banking sector reforms must continue. The major objective must be to improve the efficiency of the functioning of banks and other institutions. The recapitalization of banks and regulation of bad debts must get priority. The reform measures announced recently by the government, such as private operations in coal mining, are truly in the spirit of liberalization. They need to be implemented with dedication and commitment.

India's Growth Prospects

Many national and international agencies have projected a sharp contraction in 2020–21, ranging from (-)3.2 per cent[9] to (-)6.8 per cent. It was felt at one time that the outcome may be better than these strong contractionary projections because some key sectors, such as agriculture and related sectors, public administration, defence services, and other services may perform normally or better than normal, given the demand for health, relief and revival expenditures. We had even expected that a small positive growth might be possible. The recently released national income figures for Quarter 1 of 2020–21 hold no such hope.

---

[9]World Bank. (2020, June). 'Pandemic, Recession: The Global Economy in Crisis'. Global Economic Prospects.

India's real GDP growth at (-)23.9 per cent in the first quarter of 2020–21 signalled that the fiscal year as a whole must also end up showing a contraction. Only one sector showed positive growth on the gross value added (GVA) side, namely, agriculture. On the demand side as well, only one segment, namely, government final consumption expenditure, showed positive growth. Thus, from both demand and supply sides, the Indian economy has contracted comprehensively. This outcome has been largely due to the extensive lockdown from April 2020 onwards. The high magnitude of contraction could have been moderated, if there had been a substantial net fiscal stimulus. The fact that the GVA sector called 'public administration, defence and other services' contracted, at (-)10.3 per cent in the first quarter of 2020–21, is indicative of a weak net fiscal stimulus. The central as well as state governments and the public sector entities may all have contributed to this. In fact, the central government had frozen dearness allowance and dearness relief, and many state governments, in addition, even held back due salary payments. In order to reverse this strong contractionary trend, apart from opening up the economy, we need a substantive second round of fiscal stimulus. The financing of such a stimulus is constrained by the performance of the Centre's gross tax revenues, which have shown a contraction of more than 29 per cent in the first four months of 2020–21. As indicated earlier, a combined fiscal deficit of 12 per cent of GDP is inevitable and needed, and may have to be met by monetizing debt to a certain extent and raising resources from external sources.

In order to ensure that the Indian economy turns around in at least 2021–22, the combined fiscal deficit of the central and state governments may have to be relatively high in 2021–22 as well, as compared to the Fiscal Responsibility and Budget Management (FRBM) norms. We may consider a combined fiscal deficit of 9 per cent of GDP in 2021–22, keeping 5 per cent for the central government and 4 per cent for the state governments, so as to smoothen the path of adjustment. The emphasis on infrastructure investment should be continued in line with the investment plan for the NIP. Subsequently, a path of adjustment may need to be worked out to bring the central and state fiscal deficits in line with the FRBM norms.

Conclusion

The story of the Indian economy as it unfolds under the impact of COVID-19 is disquieting. Had the economy been strong to start with, the situation would have been different. The lockdown imposed to curb the spread of COVID-19 has put a brake on the economy. The need to kick-start the economy and move it forward has become urgent. We have, in this context, discussed the roles of monetary and fiscal policies. Maintenance of government expenditure at a high level and monetization of debt are both unavoidable. But policymakers must also be conscious of the fact that there is a limit to monetization. Wisdom lies in striking the appropriate balance.

References

Asian Development Bank. (2020, June). 'Lockdown, Loosening, and Asia's Growth Prospects'. Asian Development Outlook 2020 Supplement.

Government of India. (2020, May). 'Presentation of details of 5th Tranche announced by Union Finance and Corporate Affairs Minister Smt. Nirmala Sitharaman under Aatmanirbhar Bharat Abhiyaan to support Indian economy in fight against COVID-19'. *https://pib.gov.in/PressReleasePage.aspx?PRID=1624651*; https://static.pib.gov.in/WriteReadData/userfiles/Aatma%20Nirbhar%20Bharat%20%20Presentation%20Part%205%2017-5-2020.pdf.

Ministry of Finance. (2020, April). Government of India. 'National

Infrastructure Pipeline-Volume I'; https://dea.gov.in/sites/default/files/Report%20of%20the%20Task%20Force%20National%20Infrastructure%20Pipeline%20%28NIP%29%20-%20volume-i_1.pdf.

Ministry of Finance. (2020, April). Government of India. 'National Infrastructure Pipeline-Volume II'; https://dea.gov.in/sites/default/files/Report%20of%20the%20Task%20Force%20National%20Infrastructure%20Pipeline%20%28NIP%29%20-%20volume-ii_1.pdf.

OECD. (2020, June). 'The world economy on a tightrope'. OECD Economic Outlook 2020.

C. Rangarajan and D.K. Srivastava. (2019, August 23). 'Increasing Investment to Stimulate Growth.' *The Hindu*; https://www.thehindu.com/opinion/lead/increasing-investment-to-stimulate-growth/article29224925.ece.

Reserve Bank of India. (2020, April 17). 'Governor's statement'; https://rbidocs.rbi.org.in/rdocs/Content/PDFs/GOVERNOR STATEMENTF22E618703AE48A4 B2F6EC4A 8003F 88D. PDF.

Reserve Bank of India. 'Handbook of Statistics on Indian Economy (online)'.

Reserve Bank of India. 'Monthly Bulletin (various issues, online versions)'.

Reserve Bank of India. (2020, May 8). 'Revised Issuance Calendar for Marketable Dated Securities for the remaining period of H1 - May 11 - September 30, 2020'; https://www.rbi.org.in/Scripts/BS_Press Release Display.aspx?prid=49792.

Reserve Bank of India. (2020, March 27). 'Seventh Bi-monthly Monetary Policy Statement, 2019-20 Resolution of the Monetary Policy Committee'; https://www.rbi.org.in/Scripts/BS_Press Release Display.aspx?prid=49581.

Reserve Bank of India. (2020, February 6). 'Sixth Bi-monthly Monetary Policy Statement, 2019-20 Resolution of the Monetary Policy Committee'; https://www.rbi.org.in/Scripts/BS_Press Release Display.aspx? prid=49342.

Reserve Bank of India. (2020, May 22). 'Statement on Developmental and

Regulatory Policies'; https://www.rbi.org.in/Scripts/BS_Press Release Display.aspx? prid=49844.

Reserve Bank of India. (2020, May 20-22). 'Monetary Policy Statement, 2020-21: Resolution of the Monetary Policy Committee' https://www.rbi.org.in/Scripts/BS_PressReleaseDisplay.aspx? prid=49843.

◆

C. Rangarajan is the former governor, Reserve Bank of India, and former chairman, PMEAC, India. He was a professor at the Indian Institute of Management, Ahmedabad, and chairman, Madras School of Economics.

D.K. Srivastava is chief policy advisor, EY, and honorary professor, Madras School of Economics (MSE). He was earlier director, MSE. He has been a member of the Twelfth Finance Commission. He was also professor, National Institute for Public Finance and Policy, Delhi.

FROM A TAILSPIN TO A CRASH: WHAT NEEDS TO BE DONE

Subramanian Swamy

The Myth: 'Vikas' Since 2014

Since 2014, the Narendra Modi-led union government has announced economic objectives (i.e., made promises) in a random unstructured way, *without* stating the economic priorities. It has also outlined a strategy for achieving these objectives, and laid out measures for mobilization of the required resources.

For example, the PM announced in the last week of May of 2019, after the Bharatiya Janata Party (BJP) received a bigger mandate than in 2014, that the economy's size as measured by the GDP would double, rising from $2.5 trillion to $5 trillion, little realizing that it implied a growth rate of 14.4 per cent per year, which was then, and now even more, inconsistent with the ground realities of the economy.

In the first quarter of FY20, for example, the GDP growth rate according to an official publication was a mere 3.1 per cent on an annual basis.[10] Where is 14.4 per cent, and where will 3.1 per cent take the economy? Couldn't anyone inform the PM of this simple arithmetic, that under the prevailing circumstances, even before the coronavirus pandemic, doubling of the GDP was an impossible target that he should not speak of again?

---

[10]Government of India. (2020, June 30). Ministry of Finance, *Macroeconomic Report*.

But no one did! The PM thus repeated several times since then this presently impossible target that he was committed to achieving, till the pandemic gripped the nation and a lockdown was declared by him on 25 March—which was at the end of FY19. Modi has made other such unrealistic announcements, e.g., doubling the agricultural income in a four-year period starting 2018 (which requires an 18 per cent growth rate annually). A reality check is now in order.

The Reality: Economic Growth in Decline

Available statistical indices reveal that the Indian economy has been on a tailspin, falling into a serious crisis since FY2016; i.e., pre-COVID-19. Post-COVID, the decline or deceleration has been catastrophic, leading to negative growth rates. Chart 1 shows it vividly:

Chart 1: Estimates quarterly data on GDP growth rates, 2012–19

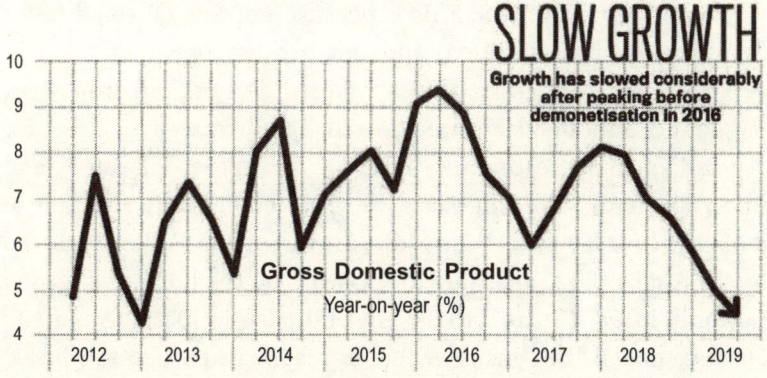

Source: Ministry of Statistics and Programme Implementation based on constant 2011–12 prices

The Modi government now admits belatedly that the revised data shows a sharp yearly fall in the GDP growth rate to 3.1 per cent in the last (fourth) quarter of 2019–20.[11] This pre-COVID-19 growth rate is less than the disparaging Hindu Rate of Growth of 3.5 per cent per year during the 1950–90 period! No spin can hide that. The latest data for the first quarter of 2020–21, i.e., April–July 2020, shows a further steep decline in GDP growth into negative digits. Predictions galore for the fiscal year 2020–21 range from the Ministry of Finance's (-)4.5 per cent to (-)15 per cent by international agencies.[12]

The pre-pandemic sectoral growth rates had also been declining across the board since 2015, and now are alarmingly negative since the coronavirus descended upon us.[13] However, the international trade and finances of India, for which we have recent data, has to be cautiously interpreted since these figures are a difference of two numbers.

Statistics put out by the RBI show that net foreign exchange earned between 1 April 2020 and 14 August 2020 has risen by $535 billion, which is 12.6 per cent above the net earnings during the same period in 2019. This is because imports declined faster than exports had declined, and not because of an increase in exports. Thus, foreign trade also suffered during the coronavirus pandemic, although net foreign exchange increased.

India's macroeconomic outlook is 'more subdued and uncertain than in recent years', the IMF euphemistically said in its latest country report on India. However, the RBI announced on 25 August 2020 that due to COVID-19, the GDP will shrink not only in Q1 (1 April to 31 July) but also in Q2 (1 August to 30 November). The consumer economy appears particularly bleak, with vehicle sales growth losing momentum. At the same time, the

---

[11] Ibid., p. 29, para 35.
[12] Ibid.
[13] Ibid., pp. 17 to 24, paras 9 to 21.

decline in tractor sales worsened. Domestic air passenger growth shows some signs of improvement but it still remains in the red.

To date, the Modi tenure's growth rate is insufficient to reduce unemployment, leave alone create full employment and reduce poverty in the country. The finance ministers of the National Democratic Alliance (NDA) government have been clueless and used the euphoria of the electoral victory of 2014 to spin the 'achievements', and since 24 March 2020, the 'green shoots' have been visible only to the ministry.

However, the reality is that the Indian economy today needs to grow at an average of 10-plus per cent per year for the next 10 years to achieve full and adequate employment, to decimate poverty, and for India to be positioned to overtake China, thus paving the way to stabilize world economy by forming a global economic bonding of India with the US. Nothing short of a growth rate of 10 per cent per year for a decade can recover India's position on the global scene, with substantial reduction in unemployment and sufficient reduction in poverty levels.

To raise GDP growth rate to more than 10 per cent, the rate of investment has to rise to 38 per cent of GDP from the present 30 per cent. Of this, household saving is the bulk of India's national investment. But since 2016, household saving has dropped from a high of 34 per cent of GDP in 2014 to 28 per cent of GDP in 2018, mainly due to the poorly implemented policies such as demonetization and low fixed deposit rate of return.

Household saving has to be incentivized (such as by abolition of personal income tax) for it to rise back to 34 per cent of GDP. Non-household saving is today about 5 per cent of GDP. For fixed deposits in banks, the rate of interest should not be less than 9 per cent per year, and this will boost personal and institutional savings in fixed deposits.

The growth rate in GDP is calculated as equal to the rate of total investment (as a ratio of GDP) divided by the productivity coefficient of capital (called incremental capital–output ratio), presently at an inefficient high of 4.5. Therefore, to achieve a 10-plus per cent growth rate in GDP, a household saving rate of 34 per cent of GDP, a non-household saving rate of 5 per cent of GDP and an incremental capital–output ratio of not more than 3.9 is necessary. That is, if the rate of investment is 39 per cent and productivity (incremental capital–output) ratio is 3.9, then GDP growth rate is equal to 39 divided by 3.9, which equals 10 per cent.

Thus, higher the productivity in the use of capital (i.e., the lower is the capital–output ratio), higher is the GDP growth rate for the same level of investment. The decline in the level of household saving thus causes a decline in the GDP growth rate and it is this issue that we must address in a future Budget, but have not done so in any of the last six Budgets in a serious way.

Since the end of 2016, there were certain economic measures, badly implemented by the Ministry of Finance, which caused a setback to the economy. The principal measures were: (a) Demonetization; (b) GST; and (c) the Insolvency and Bankruptcy Code (IBC). The economy, however, needs about $1 trillion investment in infrastructure to render Make in India a reality, but the actual investment in sanctioned projects is valued even less in real terms than the amount invested in the pre-2014 years.

The Ministry of Finance has brutally cut allocations year after year of the real investments in infrastructure despite the urgent need for such infrastructure. The manufacturing sector, especially MSMEs, which provide the bulk of the employment for the skilled and semi-skilled in the labour force, has been growing at abysmally low rates, between 2 per cent and 5 per cent. To remedy this, the interest rates on loans to MSMEs should not be more than 9 per cent—ideally at no more than 4 per cent. At present, MSMEs are lucky if loans can be got for less than 14 per cent.

India's agricultural products are among the cheapest in the world, and despite a low yield per hectare, we are not able to increase the yield to its maximum potential, or grow more than one crop per year, when in fact there are three seasons available, and thereby at least double or triple the production, and export the agricultural products abroad commensurately. Consequently, although the agriculture sector is the largest employer of India's manpower, it is grossly underperforming. Measures such as doubling incomes by doles or writing off debts are ad hoc and not long term or structural. Problems in agriculture will thus continue to recur.

While crude oil prices have steeply fallen over the four years since 2014, and despite the dollar value of the rupee remaining steadily at around ₹65 per dollar till mid-2018, *both* exports and imports have declined over the three years, 2014–17. As stated earlier, the Ministry of Finance claims to have reduced the current account deficit (CAD) in the balance of payments (BoP) accounts!

As India struggles through the coronavirus pandemic-led economic downturn, the road ahead may have more bumps as lakhs of jobs may get washed away in the next three months (as of August 2020). About 41 lakh youth may lose jobs in the next three months due to the ongoing disruptions in business activities. Over the next six months, job losses for the youth may equal 2 lakh crore in India.[14] The highest impact is expected to be seen in the construction and MSME sectors. An International Labour Organization (ILO)–Asian Development Bank report shows that youth (15–24 years) working ad hoc, such as in roadside dhabas, will be hit harder than adults (25 and older)

---

[14]Samrat Sharma, (2020, August 18). '41 lakh youth may lose jobs in 3 months', *Financial Express*, Accessed at: https://www.financialexpress.com/economy/41-lakh-youth-may-lose-jobs-in-3-months-indias-economic-woes-dont-seem-to-be-ending-soon/2058880/

in the immediate crisis.[15] These negative trends will continue *unless* the unstructured, uninformed economic 'policy' of the Modi government changes to a structured policy based on the realities of today and a recognition of the follies of the past, i.e., if the economy is not to become irretrievably stunted.

Another indicator of an embedded crisis carrying over into the post-COVID period is the admission in the 2020–21 Budget, presented on 1 February 2020, which clearly shows that the loans to be taken by the government in the Budget will almost be equal to the amount to be repaid as amortization of loans taken in the past years. In other words, even before COVID hit, we were *already* on the verge of a budgetary debt crisis—which is dangerous. Nor was there any concrete proposal in the Budget for liquidating the NPAs' burden on public sector banks. This has now become much worse. No wonder, on 26 August 2020 the Supreme Court came down heavily on the Ministry of Finance for being clueless about how to handle this.

During the lockdown, wholesale markets were open only intermittently and the cost of transporting the produce to cities has shot up. Farmers are running around with vegetables to find a buyer, leaving tomatoes to rot in the field and dumping white pumpkins by the roadside. Between April and July, as the COVID-19 pandemic worsened across India, farmers incurred heavy losses as most vegetables had to be sold for less than ₹5 per kg. Ex-farm prices were so low that they did not even cover the cost of plucking and transport. Strangely, at the consumer end of the food supply pipeline, prices have been soaring. Pulses are rare; fruits are a luxury. Consumer price index (CPI) shot up to 6.9 per cent in July driven by higher food prices, which rose 9.6 per cent year on year.

---

[15] *Tackling the COVID-19 Youth Employment Crisis in Asia and the Pacific*. (2020, August). Asian Development Bank, Manila, Accessed at: https://www.adb.org/publications/covid-19-youth-employment-crisis-asia-pacific

The pandemic has widened the gap between consumer price and ex-farm and ex-factory price to high levels. The CPI food basket shows that the increase in retail prices is on account of the rising price of cereals (7 per cent), meat and fish (19 per cent), pulses (16 per cent), vegetables (11 per cent) and edible oils (12 per cent). The high 'protein' inflation, reflecting in higher prices of meat, eggs and pulses, at a time when the pandemic has led to a sharp fall in household incomes, is indicative of continuing supply disruptions and intermediaries, using the pandemic as an excuse to jack up consumer prices.

Despite India being in 'unlock' mode, supply chains are far from normal—frequent shutdown of local wholesale and retail markets are taking a toll on primary producers. Consumers, particularly from lower income groups, are already struggling to put food on the plate.

What Needs to Be Done

Until normalcy returns, it is not appropriate to be concerned with constructing a long-term structured policy. However, for the present, till the pandemic vanishes, the government needs to focus on the human distress caused by COVID-19. This has to be first addressed by non-market government intervention. A ₹21 trillion package was announced with great fanfare, but only ₹1.5 trillion was specifically marked for direct monetary stimulus. This is disappointing. The remainder of the package is in terms of fiscal concessions for loan repayments, etc. This has had minimal impact. Moreover, the loan moratorium announced at the beginning of the pandemic by the RBI was a temporary suspension of the required EMI payments against term loans.

It is going to cause misery, especially to small traders, businesses and those of the salaried class whose jobs have been terminated because of COVID-19. There is no relief promised by the government so far. That is why the Supreme Court criticized the union government in August 2020. The Bench tersely said, according to media reports, 'This happened because you locked down the entire country'. And added: 'Don't hide behind the Reserve Bank of India'.

Nevertheless, the Modi government has distributed grains to the landless labour and cash payments to migrant daily wage workers in many states, which has given some relief. However, the government must seriously address several priority problems. It is essential to implement a new menu of measures to uplift by: (a) introducing dramatic incentives for the household expectation and sentiment to save, (b) lowering the cost of capital via reducing the prime lending interest rates of banks to 9 per cent, (c) shifting to a fixed exchange rate regime of ₹50 per dollar for FY21 and then gradually lowering the exchange rate for subsequent years to ₹10 per dollar.

Thus, the present possibility of an economic crash should galvanize us to honestly review the way we have governed and done the business of governing, and then rise to new heights by an appropriate change in policy, thereby achieving higher growth rates of 10-plus per cent annual growth in GDP with structural changes.

The BJP government also needs to give an alternative ideological thrust to economic policy rather than trying to improve on the past failed economic policies of the United Progressive Alliance (UPA), as is being done since 2014. The government should consider the following principles:

(a) The individual has to be persuaded by the government with incentives and not by coercion. Of course, the state should make no promise to the people without specifying the sacrifice required to be made by the people to make it happen.

(b) India can make rapid economic progress to become a developed country only through a globally competitive economy, which requires assured access to the markets and technological innovations of the US and some of its allies such as Israel. This has concomitant political obligations that must be accepted as essential.

Since 2016, the Indian economy has been in a steady decline, which I have previously termed as a 'tailspin'.[16] The tailspin is now headed dangerously close to a crash. The good news is that the current developing crisis does not necessarily mean an irreversible collapse of the Indian economy. In the last 73 years, India has always come out of crises once these were acknowledged and then dealt with, without resorting to a self-deluding spin.

As examples, I can cite the food crisis of 1965–67, on which foreign scholars predicted a massive famine, but which instead led to the Green Revolution and food self-sufficiency. When I had just become commerce minister, the foreign exchange crisis of 1990–91 led to economic reforms. This contributed to higher GDP growth rates during PM Narasimha Rao's tenure, rising from a 3.5 per cent annual trend rate of four decades (1950–80) to 8.5 per cent by 1995–96.

The situation of crisis in the Indian economy today is also retrievable, and a turnaround can be achieved within three months after certain 'real' economic policy changes. To seriously address the current priority problems, it is essential to implement the following menu of new measures to uplift economic growth:

(a) Provide dramatic incentives for the households to spend and for the sentiment to save, by measures such as the abolition of personal income tax

---

[16] Subramanian Swamy. (2015, September 18). 'The Way Out of the Economic Tailspin', *The Hindu*, Accessed at: https://www.thehindu.com/opinion/lead/the-way-out-of-the-economic-tailspin/article7662610.ece

(b) Lower the cost of capital by reducing the prime lending interest rates of banks to 9 per cent
(c) Shift to a fixed exchange rate regime of ₹35 per dollar for FY20 and then gradually lowering the exchange rate for subsequent years to what is the purchasing power parity (PPP) rate of ₹7 per dollar
(d) Print adequate rupee notes to fully finance basic infrastructure projects while keeping concerns about fiscal deficit ratio in the cold storage
(e) Invoke the UN Resolution of 2005 on Corruption to bring back black money of about $1 trillion stashed abroad, and held illegally; and
(f) Abolish Participatory Notes while invoking the UN Resolution of 2005 to bring back the $1 trillion illegal black money, and printing rupee notes to fully finance basic infrastructure projects while keeping concerns about fiscal deficit ratio for the time being in the cold storage.

The impending threat of an economic crash should galvanize the government to honestly review the way we have governed in the past and brought the economy to this sad state. Policy should be structured around specific objectives, with implied targets for investment, employment and productivity, based on a clear understanding of macroeconomics and not on spins such as 'green shoots'. While India has demonstrated impressive prowess in IT, biotechnology, automobile ancillaries and pharmaceuticals, and had also accelerated its growth rate since 1991 to become the third largest nation in terms of GDP at PPP rates, it still has a backward agricultural sector, employing 62 per cent of the labour force, where farmers are ending their lives unable to repay their loans, with an inefficient use of a large investment level that largely depends on high household savings as a ratio of GDP.

The Indian economy is also saddled with a national unemployment rate, which is now over 25 per cent of the adult labour force, a prevalence of child labour arising out of nearly 50 per cent of children not making it to school beyond Standard V, a deeply malfunctioning primary and secondary educational system, 300 million illiterates and 250 million people in a dire state of poverty.

Moreover, India's educated youth is skill-deficient, risk-averse in attitude and largely unemployable in the cutting-edge manufacturing sector. As per a plan outlined in Macaulay's Minute on Education (1835), our universities still produce clerks for government administration or employers for the corporate sector and not risk-taking innovators of the future, who'll raise the productivity of capital and labour. Although a New Education Policy 2020 has been presented, it is in the form of recommendations, and will have to be presented before the Parliament as bills and claims on the Budget in the form of appropriations.

India's infrastructure is in a pathetic state, with frequent power breakdowns even in metropolitan cities, a dangerously unhealthy water supply system in urban areas and a very poor road network with gaping holes even on national highways. The infrastructure sector requires at least about $1 trillion to make it world-class, while the education system needs 6 per cent of GDP instead of the 2.8 per cent today.

These problems can be addressed only by a comprehensive, second-generation, systemic reform that makes the economy an efficient, competitive, market-oriented one, which leverages our potentialities (such as our civilizational heritage of innovative intellect) and minimizes the inefficiency, squandering and corruption in the deployment of our vast resources. India has much potential today to become a booming economy: it has a demographic dividend of a young population with an average

age of 28 years compared to China's 35 years, the US's 38 years, Europe's 46 years and Japan's 49 years. Internationally, Indian agriculture has the lowest yield in land and livestock-based milk products, whose yield can easily be raised judging by the performance in experimental agricultural plots of the Indian Agricultural Research Institute and the Indian Council of Agricultural Research, and also by borrowing agricultural techniques from Israel.

India's cost of production for agriculture and milk production is low when compared internationally. With proper infrastructure and packaging, India can certainly become a global player in agricultural exports. Even though India is also gifted with a full 12 months-a-year of farm-friendly weather, it grows just one crop a year in over 75 per cent of arable land, when it can grow three crops. It also has the advantage of a highly competitive, skilled labour force and low wage rates at the national level, the advantages of which have been already proved to the world by the outsourcing phenomenon. What is needed is a bold commitment of sufficient resources to harvest this potential.

An open competitive market system can find these resources from non-tax sources, as has been demonstrated in the auction of the 2G Spectrum licences following the Supreme Court judgment on my Special Leave Petition in 2012. A transparent policy regime, auctioning of natural resources (if it is used for a commercial private enterprise) and the unearthing of the vast $1 trillion in black money stashed abroad will enable the government to marshal sufficient resources for a massive investment in a second-generation economic reform while reducing the tax burden on people.

If the quality of governance and accountability is improved, then the incremental capital–output will also reduce, thus raising the growth rate of GDP. As an economist, the only advice I can give the Modi government is to take some steps that will raise the morale of the consumer and investor. That means income tax abolition and reducing the annual interest rate (prime lending rate) to 9 per cent.

The good news is that the built-in potential in the economy is easy to tap for revival, as is the basic resilience of the Indian people to face any situation, as demonstrated from past crises. India can rise to new heights by appropriate change in policy and governance, and thus achieve higher growth rates of 10-plus per cent annual growth in GDP with healthy structural changes for productivity-raising innovations.

Modern economic growth is powered overwhelmingly (over 65 per cent of GDP) by new innovation and techniques (e.g., internet). More capital and labour contributes less than 35 per cent of growth in GDP. India today leads the world in the supply pool of youth, i.e., persons in the age group of 15–35 years, and this lead will last for another 40 years. This generation is a most fertile milieu for promoting knowledge, innovation and research. It is the prime workforce that saves for the future, the corpus for pension-funding of the old. We should therefore not squander this natural vital resource of demographic dividend.

◆

Subramanian Swamy is a Member of Parliament. He earned his doctorate at Harvard, writing his thesis under Nobel Laureate Simon Kuznets and published a seminal joint-authored research with Nobel Laureate Paul Samuelson on Index Numbers. He has taught at the Harvard University and at the Indian Institute of Technology, Delhi. He has been a minister for Commerce and Law & Justice, Government of India.

COVID ECONOMY AND THE MAY 2020 PACKAGE

Bibek Debroy

This is not the best of times to write such an essay, when much is uncertain. Economists like precision and split hairs between uncertainty and risk. Risk is associated with known probabilities of events. Uncertainty occurs when even those probabilities are unknown. This is a period of uncertainty, not risk. We don't know when COVID-19 numbers will taper off, worldwide or in India. We don't know if there would be a second phase. With a virus that mutates, we don't know if, and when, there will be a vaccine and how it will be distributed. Yes, models are possible. But worldwide, and for India, such models on COVID-19 spread have proved to be wrong and are no longer plausible. If the trajectory of the virus is uncertain, its imprint on the economy cannot be vested with any degree of certitude.

The notion of 'recession' emerged in advanced economies. These economies achieved their present prosperous and developed status by growing at between 1 per cent and 2 per cent over several decades. Compared to recent real rates of growth in Asia, Africa and elsewhere, these are low rates. Though recession has many nuances and attributes—with between 1 per cent and 2 per cent regarded as indicative of potential—the most common definitions of recession involve declines in GDP, or negative rates of growth, over two successive quarters. Thus defined, COVID-19 has led to the deepest global recession in decades, undisputedly the largest contraction in the global economy since World War II. That statement is based on projections.

For obvious reasons, actual numbers only surface with a time lag. There are several points to note about these projections, such as growth forecasts announced by the IMF. First, progressively, over time, the forecasts continue to become worse. For instance, WEO projections in June 2020 are more sombre than those in April 2020.

Second, for the calendar year 2020, IMF's latest projections suggest a contraction in global growth by 4.9 per cent. Just so that we have the right comparative benchmarks, during the global financial crisis of 2008, global growth contracted only by 07 per cent. That's a completely different order of magnitude. A contraction of 4.9 per cent in 2020 isn't expected to be evenly spread among groups of countries. It's worse for advanced economies than for emerging markets and developing economies.

Third, in 2021, projections suggest a growth of 5.4 per cent. So that we don't get bogged down in the semantics, this is V-shaped recovery in a pedantic sense, the decline in 2020 offset by the growth in 2021. And yes, there are variations in this across groups of countries. For advanced economies, growth in 2021 doesn't quite compensate for decline in 2020, and for emerging markets and developing economies, it is just the reverse.

Fourth—and this is a crucial point—that 'V' is defined in terms of rates of growth, not in terms of absolute levels of activity. The level of global output in 2021 will be just about what it was in 2019—indeed, a little less. Without factoring in adverse longer-term effects on human development outcomes (health, education, productivity), the world will have lost two years of development. This is a stark, but true, way of stating what COVID-19 has done. The Sustainable Development Goals (SDGs) have a target date of 2030. Since that goalpost hasn't moved, the SDGs become more difficult to achieve.

China was responsible for COVID-19 and its spread, deliberately or inadvertently. It has also been responsible for non-COVID-19–related tensions, deliberately. Across a range of countries, in the middle of the pandemic, and even before it, China has exhibited its cross-border territorial ambitions, on both sea and land. The unnecessary intervention in Hong Kong's national security legislation not only raises questions about the nature of Hong Kong's autonomy, but also about Hong Kong's relationships with the rest of the world.

Security concerns and trade/investments aren't silos that exist in isolation, delinked from each other. Security concerns will inevitably lead to trade action against China, as the EU, the US and India have done. Nor should one forget that China became a member of the WTO in December 2001, with the expectation that beyond December 2016, China would introduce reforms to transit to market economy status. In December 2016, China requested consultations with the EU, alleging that it wasn't treating China as a market economy in anti-dumping and anti-subsidy investigations.

Thereafter, in July 2017, China formally complained to the WTO about the EU's action. When the panel report was ready in 2019 and about to be made public, China withdrew the complaint. Logically, this can only mean that China anticipated that the findings would be adverse. As a multilateral institution, WTO is not in the best of shape now and WTO-driven negotiations have all but collapsed, with even the dispute resolution mechanism brought into question. Stated simply, exports (more precisely, net exports) are unlikely to be a major contributor to economic growth. Both because of trade and non-trade tensions, the global environment today is malign, not benign.

Real rates of growth can be subject to year-to-year fluctuations. If one looks beyond such fluctuations, there were periods when India's real rate of growth was 8 per cent or more—roughly from

2003–04 to 2010–11, and then again, roughly from 2014–15 to 2016–17. In the first of these two periods, but not in the second, global growth rates were high. India's net exports (exports minus imports) performed well and India's trade/GDP ratio increased. Trade was a driver of economic growth.

There is a national income identity: $Y = C + I + G + (X-M)$. Since it is an identity, it must definitionally always be true. There can only be four sources of growth: (1) consumption; (2) investments; (3) government expenditure; and (4) net exports. From what has been said, net exports get knocked out as a source of growth. As was the case during the period from 2014–15 to 2016–17, sources of growth will have to be endogenous: C, I and G.

If one leaves out railways and defence, and of course union territories, an all-India rate of growth is a function of the GSDP growth rates, aggregated upwards. Beyond year-to-year fluctuations again, states such as Gujarat, Andhra Pradesh, Haryana and Madhya Pradesh have clocked 8 per cent and more real rates of growth for more than a single year, but most other states have not. If those lagging states manage to jack up their rates of growth, we can presumably do 8 per cent at an all-India level. Thus, 8 per cent is something like a potential rate of growth. To reiterate, India achieved that 8 per cent between 2014–15 and 2016–17. As was mentioned, this was a period when world growth didn't perform that well. Therefore, even though world growth will remain lacklustre in the immediate future, 8 per cent should be doable. There is enough endogenous slack to achieve that.

Where do we stand now? There are a range of projections for growth in 2020–21. Broadly, they suggest a negative growth rate of between 5 per cent and 7 per cent. The growth performance would have been worse had it not been for agriculture. For 2020–21, Q3 and Q4 will be better than Q1 and Q2, and there are some indicators that show a revival of activity to almost pre-COVID and pre-lockdown levels, partly a reflection of pent-up demand.

In parallel, there are projections for 2021–22, suggesting positive growth of between 6 per cent and 8 per cent. Not surprisingly, for 2021–22, projected growth rates are higher for Q1 and Q2 than for Q3 and Q4. The reason is obvious. Once one understands that, they should appreciate that the discourse over a V-shaped recovery for India is also pointless, as it is for the world. The reason for this recovery is statistical, because of the low base in 2020–21. If one plots a trajectory across quarters, growth rates in 2021–22 will be a mirror image of growth rates in 2020–21. The lower it was in 2020–21, the higher it will be in 2021–22 and so on.

This recovery is in growth rates not in the absolute level, and there is an important difference between the two. The right question to ask is the following: What will be the absolute level of GDP at the beginning of 2022–23, compared to that at the end of 2019–20? They will probably be just about the same. Indeed, at the beginning of 2022–23 it may be a little bit lower, since COVID-19 may have left adverse effects on labour and productivity.

Stated differently, we have lost two years of development because of the pandemic. There was a target about the size of India's economy becoming a $5 trillion figure by 2024–25. The size of the economy is just short of $3 trillion now. This is a 2019 figure, from World Bank sources. That's the base from which one hopes to achieve the $5 trillion aspirational target. Estimating the real rate of growth required to achieve the $5 trillion target by 2024–25 depends on assumptions made, both about the rate of inflation and the exchange rate. Depending on the assumptions—and there is no reason for the rupee to appreciate significantly against the US dollar over this short time frame—the required real rate of growth will be around 8.5 per cent.

Because of the way recession is defined, the phrase 'growth recession' is an oxymoron, despite it being used indiscriminately by commentators and media. When the potential is 1 per cent to

2 per cent, which it was for advanced economies, a negative rate of growth, illustrated in the way recession came to be defined, is a red flag. When the potential is 8 per cent, which is what it should be for India, by the same token, anything below 6 per cent should be a red flag for India. Though one should not use the expression 'growth recession' for technical reasons, the moment real growth drops below 6 per cent, one should worry.

The dropping of real growth to below 6 per cent predates COVID-19. A progressive decline in growth over quarters became especially sharp in 2019–20. An explanation as to why this occurred helps shape a future course of action. Decomposed as C, I and G, the growth between 2014–15 and 2016–17 was primarily driven by consumption and government expenditure, not by investments—or to use the right expression, gross fixed capital formation. In ensuring the revival of growth from 2022–23 and ensuring an increase from 6 per cent to 8 per cent or thereabouts, investments will remain the key.

Growth and GDP aren't mere numbers; they have implications for poverty and employment. In a largely informal and unorganized economy, even outside agriculture, in the absence of proper household surveys, data on both poverty and employment is unreliable. Unfortunately, the last such reliable survey was undertaken by the National Sample Survey Office (NSSO) in 2011–12. Because of COVID-19, the next consumption survey by NSSO will be delayed to 2021–22 and beyond.

Poverty is a multidimensional concept. However, it has been traditionally estimated as a poverty ratio, the percentage of population below a poverty line. Though there are subsequent World Bank sources for such numbers, the last national poverty estimate was for 2011–12, when the national poverty ratio was 21.9 per cent, with expected variations among states and poverty more concentrated in some states than in others.

The SDGs have a terminal timeline of 2030. There is a diverse template of goals, targets and indicators, and India has its own national indicator framework. In terms of this, the intended poverty rate in 2030 is expected to be 10.95 per cent. COVID-19 makes it a bit more difficult to achieve this, not merely because we have lost two years of development. Temporally, India's poverty rate has declined, but that decline hasn't been linear over time. That's because income and consumption distributions are typically log normal. When the thick part of the distribution passes above the designated poverty line, as the distribution shifts to the right because of growth, sharp non-linear drops in poverty are seen. If there is an adverse and exogenous shock, sharp increases in poverty are also possible. Poverty numbers drop because individuals/households who are just below the poverty line have risen above it. With a shock, they can drop below the poverty line again.

The poverty ratio was just one example. The same logic also applies to the other SDGs/indicators. Achieving them in 2030 becomes more difficult. Take for instance, savings. Since 2011–12, when the new GDP series was started, it isn't merely the investment rate (as a share of GDP) that has declined, the savings rate has declined too. If one breaks up savings into its three components of households, private corporate and public, the savings decline has been marked for the household sector. With the consequences of both COVID-19-related health expenditure and lockdown-related livelihood issues, have households dipped into their financial savings and will the savings rate decline further, at least in the immediate short term? We don't have data, but it is a concern.

However, it is also true that without government interventions since 2014, India would have fared worse under COVID-19, although at one level, this remains a counter-factual argument. Without getting into details, as that will be too much of a digression, examples of such interventions are the Mahatma

Gandhi National Rural Employment Guarantee Act (MGNREGA), Pradhan Mantri Jan-Dhan Yojana (PMJDY), National Social Assistance Programme, Housing for All, Saubhagya, Pradhan Mantri Jan Arogya Yojana, Ayushman Bharat, Swachh Bharat Abhiyan, direct benefit transfer (DBT) and Aadhaar. Rural India was relatively insulated from both COVID-19 and the lockdown. But, in addition, rural India has benefited more from public welfare schemes, facilitated by the Socio-Economic Caste Census (SECC) (rural) being more robust than SECC (urban). For rural India, there has been a better and easier matching of household identification (such as in MGNREGA and SECC), with individual identification (such as in Ayushman Bharat and Aadhaar). If there was a problem with urban migrants returning to rural India, it was largely because the identification requirement of the Inter-State Migrant Workmen Act of 1979 was never implemented, and welfare benefits lacked portability.

Between 13 May and 17 May 2020, the finance minister announced an economic reform package in five tranches. One of the items mentioned was the portability of ration cards, to be completed throughout the country by March 2021. The eventual goal is portability that extends to all welfare schemes, not just ration cards. There is a double identity problem one should be aware of. First, India still lacks a national identity for individuals. Yes, significant financial inclusion has been accomplished through PMJDY, and in many instances these have been linked to Aadhaar numbers. For pensions, scholarships and now the health schemes, there can be direct transfers to these bank accounts. However, targeting of beneficiaries is often household-based (MGNREGA, SECC). The household-to-individual matching has to be done and is still work in progress, a trend now accentuated because of COVID-19 and the focus on health. Second, unincorporated enterprise also lacks identity, though a GST network provides a working base. For instance, most MSMEs have no legal identity, not having been set up under any statutory law. Therefore, any government initiative (credit, equity, government procurement) only benefits the top layer of MSMEs. Both identity problems are reflective of a transition from an informal to a formal economy. No such transition occurs overnight. However, COVID-19, and more importantly, the lockdown, act as an exogenous shock to catalyze the process, evident in the faster pace of digitization.

The May economic reform package was criticized because the government had not done enough, in terms of direct fiscal expenditure. After all, as we argued earlier, sources of growth will have to be C, I and G. But on that G, several points need to be made: First, when arguing in favour of expansionary fiscal policy, more often than not, expectations are about reduced taxes, on the personal income tax side and the corporate side. Are these sector-specific? If they are, they distort resource allocation and make the task of tax reform, which involves standardization and simplification, more difficult.

Second, if they aren't sector-specific but across the board, the corporate tax rate, without exemptions, is either 15 per cent or 22 per cent. Without exemptions, personal income tax rates are 10 per cent, 15 per cent and 20 per cent for different income slabs. Neither the corporate rates, nor the personal income ones, are inordinately high. They are high only if one opts for exemptions. Note that agricultural income is not taxed, even above a threshold, and this happens to be a state subject.

Third, when the GST was introduced, the revenue neutral average GST rate was expected to be at least 16 per cent. Thanks to many items in the exempted and 5 per cent brackets, it is around 11.5 per cent now. The upshot of all this is that a substantive tax reform (removal of exemptions) will involve an increase in the effective tax rate, not a reduction. But obviously, COVID-19 and its aftermath is not the best of times to implement this.

Fourth, both theoretical and empirical literature indicate that expenditure multipliers are superior to tax multipliers. In other words, expansionary fiscal policy needs to be construed as increase in public expenditure, not tax reductions.

Fifth, while fiscal deficits need not be a fetish, there are fiscal constraints on increasing public expenditure. If the nominal rate of growth is low, it has implications for government revenue, both union and states. If the nominal rate of growth is lower than the rate at which the government borrows, there is a problem with managing government debt, and beyond 2021–22 there will have to be a credible trajectory for reducing the debt/GDP ratio.

Sixth, the question, therefore, isn't simply one of increasing public expenditure, but reprioritizing it (such as towards health) and increasing its efficiency, such as a review of centrally sponsored schemes. Should there be a centrally sponsored scheme in an area that is in the State List in the Seventh Schedule? If it is important enough, why should there not be a central sector scheme, without a matching contribution from the states? Should there be a review of the Seventh Schedule? Within expenditure switching, to what extent can one switch from revenue expenditure to capital expenditure (such as infrastructure)?

Seventh, given what has been said about taxes, can one monetize public assets and drive public sector undertaking disinvestments? What constrains the National Investment Pipeline? The May economic package was criticized as not being large enough, interpreted as percentage of GDP. A comparison with other countries is irrelevant because different countries have different fiscal bases. The seven points listed above indicate that the proposition about expansionary fiscal policy is not that simple to unravel. There are complicated union–state issues to be resolved on revenue, expenditure and reform. Constitutionally, most of these are outside the Finance Commission's mandate, and the GST Council's mandate is also limited. There is a need for such a union–state forum. The historical National Development

Council was largely ornamental. In many respects, the reform template involves tweaking of the historical Government of India Act of 1935 (preceded by that of 1919) and without such a forum, that's not possible. The health crisis has emphasized this even more.

Is the National Disaster Management Act of 2005 equipped to handle emergencies and introduce uniform protocols? As of now, despite these seven points, there is scope for an additional fiscal expenditure of at least 1 per cent of GDP, perhaps even closer to 2 per cent. But the composition (with competing claims on public resources), timing and sequencing of that package would have to be right. For example, when large swathes of the country are in the midst of some sort of lockdown and there are supply-side constraints, the supply curve is inelastic. Expansionary fiscal policy does nothing to stimulate output; it merely increases prices. Government announcements have implicitly hinted that there will be another stimulus package. Other than reforms, the May package focused on credit and postponement of procedural compliances. At the time of writing this essay, the expected fiscal package is still awaited.

Before COVID-19, there was often a sterile debate about whether the growth deceleration was demand-constrained or supply-constrained. This is a sterile debate because the world is not one of binaries. As was mentioned, growth between 2014–15 and 2016–17 was primarily driven by C and G, not I. What deters investments, apart from the obvious correlation between exports and investments? If the export performance is lacklustre, especially for manufacturing, capacity-utilization levels will be low. Though the answer partly varies from sector to sector, in general, fresh investments don't occur until capacity utilization crosses a threshold, with the caveat that investments aren't a function of today's demand, but also expectations about future demand.

Given the unkind external environment, the policy question

reduces to (a) ensuring that an environment for growth and consumption increases; (b) within the fiscal constraints, increasing government expenditure such that it catalyzes I; and (c) removing policy constraints that hinder domestic and foreign investments. Interpreted thus, this is no different from supply-side reforms that commentators have spoken about. The reforms of May 2020 (amendment of Essential Commodities Act; e-trading of agricultural products; opening up minerals, defence, airspace, power distribution), part of the package the finance minister announced, should be viewed in that light. While the pandemic may have been the immediate trigger, there is continuity with reforms introduced since May 2014.

In simple terms, growth increases when the average productivity of India's citizens (at least those who are in working age groups) increases. Growth is a function of land (or natural resources), labour, capital and productivity. Other than industrial delicencing, the reforms of 1991 were primarily about border measures (exchange rate, export subsidies, quantitative restrictions, tariffs, foreign direct investment [FDI]). Post-1991, reforms are about within-border factor markets, none of which function efficiently. Reforms are about competition, and competition requires both entry and exit. Whatever be the complaints about the functioning of the IBC, the fact remains that until 2016, there was no real threat of failed entrepreneurship being forced to exit.

With labour on the Concurrent List, the union government's initiative on unifying labour laws into four codes doesn't really go far enough. Having inherited the same colonial law, Bangladesh unified all its labour laws into a single code in 2006. There is a political economy of handling union–state relations, particularly because labour conditions are not uniform throughout the country. The first National Labour Commission (NLC) was set up in the second half of the 1960s. Perhaps one needs to set up a second NLC. Land laws (not just ownership) vary widely across states, as do the quality of titling, revenue records and cadastral surveys. Land, under the Seventh Schedule, happens to be entirely a state subject. The union government's attempts at improving logistics are essentially about what happens at the border. Within-border inefficiencies are state subjects.

There was a recent (July 2020) report by TeamLease[17] on India's compliance burden. The headline that grabbed attention was that India's regulatory landscape, across union and state governments, has 1,536 acts, 69,233 compliances and 6,618 regulatory filings. This sounds horrendous. But the headlines don't mention that most are about labour, while a bulk of the remainder is about environment, health and safety. Per se, clearances aren't the problem. But rent-seeking and the consequent time taken are indeed issues, and constrain investments. After all, one requires land, forest and environment clearances.

Simplifying these has always been part of the reform agenda. With COVID-19 and lockdown, global trade and non-trade tensions, the review of trade agreements, investments vacating China and the focus on Make in India, the emphasis on reforms has been further enhanced. At the time of writing, the COVID-19 numbers look bad (more on infections and less on deaths). Being branded as the epicentre of the epidemic is not an enviable position to be in. However, with the numbers dramatically increasing in some states, it is understandable that there should be various versions of lockdown. Once life adjusts to the new normal and stabilizes, union and state governments working together should

---

[17] TeamLease Services is one of India's leading human resource companies offering a range of solutions to 3500-plus employers for their hiring, productivity and scale challenges.

R. Nair. (2020, July 08). Ease of doing business? India still has 1,536 Acts, 69,233 compliances for firms to follow. Retrieved November 10, 2020, from https://theprint.in/economy/ease-of-doing-business-india-still-has-1536-acts-69233-compliances-for-firms-to-follow/456867/

make India the epicentre of growth. There will be new ways we look at labour markets and migration. There will be new ways we look at health—morbidity and mortality. There will be new ways we look at urbanization. There will be new ways we think of India.

◆

Bibek Debroy is an economist and is currently the chairman of the PMEAC.

DESIGNING A POST-COVID RECOVERY

RAJIV KUMAR and AJIT PAI

The Context

Both tenures of the Narendra Modi government are characterized by several path-breaking reforms that had a dual objective. The first goal was to ensure that those at the bottom of the pyramid would maximally benefit from rapid economic growth as it ensued. The second goal was to make significant strides in giving greater space and momentum to private sector-led growth. Under the first goal, the set of measures included initiatives for financial inclusion, efficient delivery of public services by maximizing transfer through DBTs using the JAM trinity (Jan Dhan Yojana, Aadhaar and mobile technology), ensuring medical insurance cover for 100 million families, providing clean fuel to 120 million households, successfully implementing the Open Defecation Free programme across the country, and finally, a much-needed agricultural reform that was holding back farm workers who comprise over 40 per cent of the workforce.

Measures for promoting private enterprise and investment included improving India's ease of doing business as measured by the World Bank; implementing the historical GST, thereby integrating into a single market with easier flow of goods across state borders; ushering in the IBC, which for the first time gave creditors sufficient rights over defaulting borrowers and simplified the exit process; extensive liberalization of the FDI regime, including in defence production; taking steps for the disinvestment of central public sector enterprises deemed non-strategic to reduce distortions in the market and bringing greater efficiencies to the economy; monetization/recycling of public assets that would benefit from private participation; and simplifying 29 central labour laws into four labour codes.

The necessary cleaning up of the banking sector due to the profligate lending subsequent to the global financial crisis of 2008 and several long-overdue disruptive changes with significant long-term benefits have short-term transition costs that collectively contributed to a deceleration of economic growth. Non-farm credit growth from scheduled commercial banks (SCBs) plummeted from 24 per cent in FY11 to 5 per cent in FY20, with some sectors, such as exports and industry, suffering a net real decline

Chart 1: SCBs credit growth decelerated from 25 per cent year on year in FY11 to 5 per cent year on year in FY20, providing an average headwind of over 5 per cent annually to GDP growth

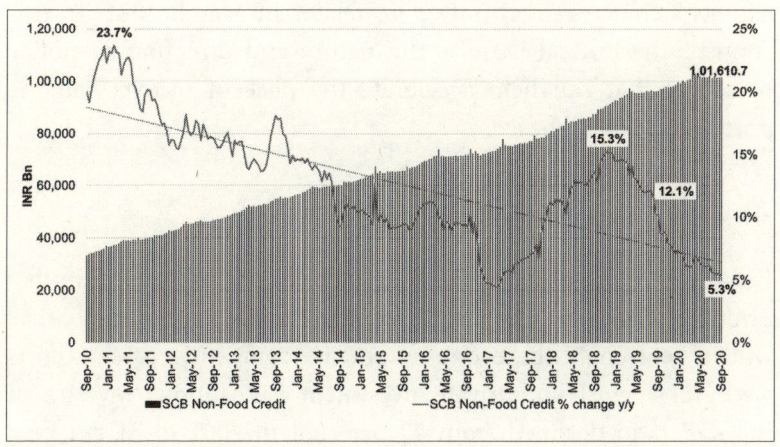

Source: RBI

in total credit outstanding, impacting the annual average growth rate of the economy by over 5 per cent. Despite these headwinds and legacy issues, average annual GDP growth from FY15 to FY20 was an impressive 6.7 per cent, and was a testimony to the positive impact of many unprecedented structural reforms undertaken during this time.

The economy was expected to reaccelerate after bottoming out in the final quarter of FY20 when GDP grew by just 3 per cent. The expectation clearly was that the strong foundations laid during the prior six years would sustain the reacceleration for several years. However, this expectation was thwarted by the onset of COVID-19, which forced a countrywide and sustained lockdown of the entire economy to prevent the pandemic from spreading at alarming rates and save precious lives. The result has been that the first quarter of FY21 saw an unprecedented decline in GDP growth of 24 per cent, with several sectors suffering a complete collapse of output, including exports and foreign tourist arrivals that were virtually stalled due to the worldwide negative impact of the pandemic. From most accounts and estimates, FY21 will see negative GDP growth, with the March 2020 level of economic activity being regained only a year later in March 2021. In this context, the critical issue is the nature and direction of policy measures that can help accelerate the pace of recovery in the post COVID-19 phase.

Approach to Post-COVID Recovery

Before getting into this critical question, it is useful to recount that prior to COVID-19, despite all the structural reforms and political will to rejuvenate the economy and its competitiveness, exports were still sluggish and private investment was cautious. Investment to GDP ratio declined from 42 per cent in 2007 to 31 per cent in 2018. Indian trade had grown rapidly subsequent to bringing

Chart 2: Priority sector credit to exporters is down by two-thirds from its peak

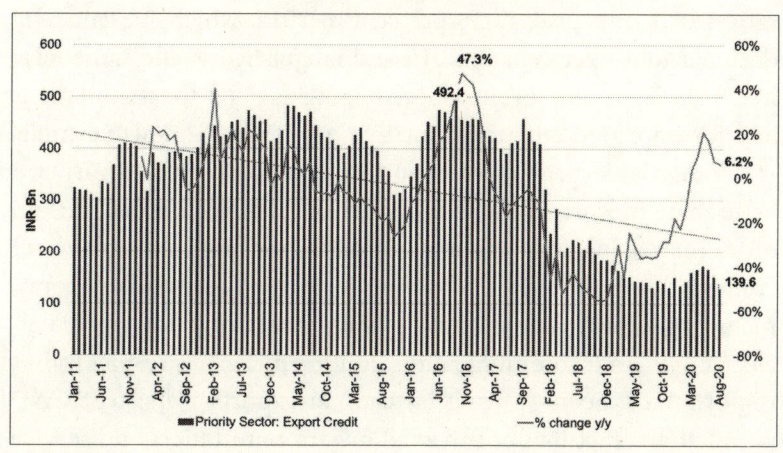

Source: RBI

Chart 3: SCB credit to industry has been stagnant in real terms over the past decade

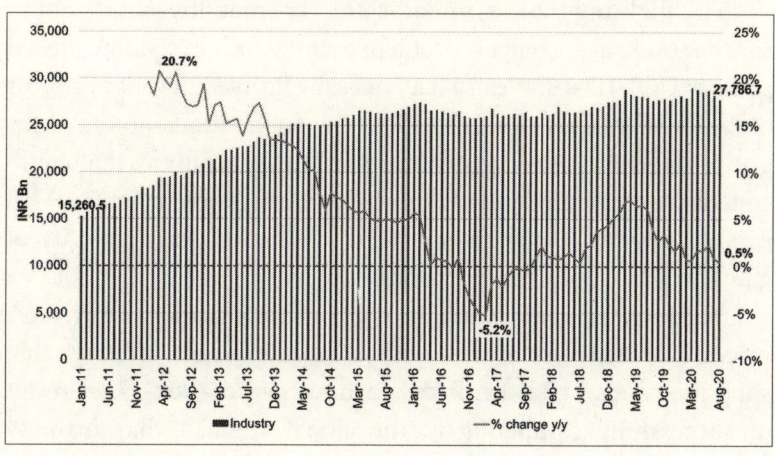

Source: RBI

down barriers steadily from the early 1990s, and solid progress to facilitate trade had been made in recent years. But the trade-to-GDP ratio reached its peak of 56 per cent in 2012, which subsequently declined to 40 per cent in 2016 and languished at the same level in 2019. There has been a decade-long lag for the foundations laid for improved competitiveness to get reflected in actual trade.

Indian enterprises and exporters have been able to garner a large share in world trade in only a few sectors. In contrast, certain economies using anti-competitive, state-sponsored strategies have come to dominate critical, enabling sectors of the global economy, including steel, aluminium, pharmaceutical intermediates, electronics and communication equipment. As a result, India's imports have been growing faster than exports. Persistent CAD points to the fact that positive net inward remittances and service exports are not sufficient or growing fast enough to compensate for the merchandise trade deficit. In contrast to East Asian economies and even the newly emerging competing countries like Vietnam and Bangladesh, India has been unable to take advantage of external demand to bolster its growth rate.

Highlighting trade as an indicator of competitiveness is not to say that trade is the biggest problem that the Indian economy faced prior to COVID-19. We use it as an easily visible relevant indicator and a benchmark to make evident the tremendous potential for greater efficiencies and growth in the Indian economy that could contribute to significantly better living conditions in India. With exports only at 19 per cent of GDP, clearly the vast majority of gains will be captured domestically.

The largest benefit would be the consumer surplus from lower prices and better products, with a more efficient industry that supplies goods at lower prices to domestic markets as a result of successfully competing in the global arena. India's inability to create large, globally competitive companies may explain a significant portion of the gap between China's and India's domestic savings and investments as proportions of their respective GDPs. Another reason to watch trade closely is that it is a powerful forward indicator for accelerating GDP growth.

Chart 4: India's and China's domestic savings and investments as percentage of GDP

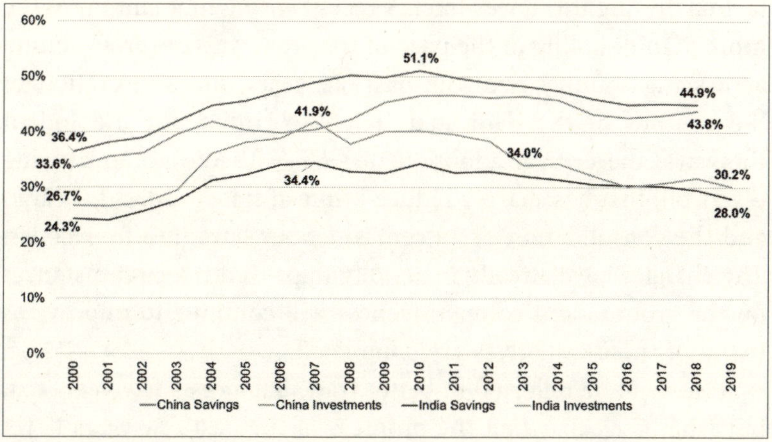

[Line chart showing China Savings, China Investments, India Savings, and India Investments from 2000 to 2019. Key data points: China Savings rises from 36.4% (2000) to peak 51.1% (around 2010), declining to 44.9% (2019). China Investments rises from 33.6% to 43.8%. India Savings starts at 26.7%, peaks at 41.9% (around 2007), declines to 28.0%. India Investments starts at 24.3%, rises to 34.4% then 34.0%, declining to 30.2%.]

Source: World Bank

The fact that must be fully digested is that China's strategy of providing universally cheaper and more reliable power and logistics for enterprises is a far more efficient driver of economic growth than handing out fiscal subsidies to exporters to make up deficiencies in these vital areas. Building a globally competitive logistics and energy sector that provides world-class services and inputs to exporters and all other domestic enterprises is far more sustainable as a growth and export strategy than trying to compensate exporters ex post facto for these gaps.

It should, however, be clearly understood that these structural drivers of competitiveness take years to be built in advance of the improvement becoming evident in increased competitiveness and rise in shares in world trade. Traders will price products and provide lead times on the basis of contemporary circumstances. But changing these circumstances, ranging from better connectivity to improved logistics, more flexible labour laws and easier/cheaper access to capital, may take years.

Once actually competitive, there is still a period of time to win market share and establish reputation. These have been the factors driving this government's recent strong momentum in the more than doubling of the pace of new road surface provisioning across the country over the past six years, the acceleration of the roll-out of the dedicated freight corridors for the Indian Railways, the critical adoption of GST with the accompanying e-way bill that has sharply reduced time at state borders for cargo and the consolidation of 29 central labour laws into four codes. The changes have already materially improved the circumstances on the ground, and competitiveness will continue to improve as many of these initiatives are completed.

This will be reflected in better trade balances a few years out, but what is clear is that the progress of the past few years is yet not sufficient to close the large competitiveness gap between India and its more efficient trading partners/competitors who have been allowed to emerge over previous decades. This also explains in large part the relatively lower benefits that have accrued to India from the bilateral and regional trade deals it has entered into over the past decade and a half. Our exporters have simply not received the logistics and input price support that their competitors take for granted in partner countries. Much more needs to be done for India to become the economic powerhouse that it has the potential to be.

It is undeniable that despite its weakness in logistics and critical inputs for exports, the opening up of India's economy to greater trade in the early 1990s significantly boosted India's GDP growth on an absolute and relative basis. India's increase in per capita GDP from about 7 per cent of the world average in

1992 to almost 19 per cent in 2019 was an impressive reversal in trajectory of previous decades when protectionism was the ruling ideology. In that protectionist era, which lasted for three decades from the 1960s to the end of the 1980s, India's per capita GDP

Chart 5 and 6: GDP per capita as percentage of world average; China has had 4x the slope as the trajectory of India in terms of improving its relative GDP per capita

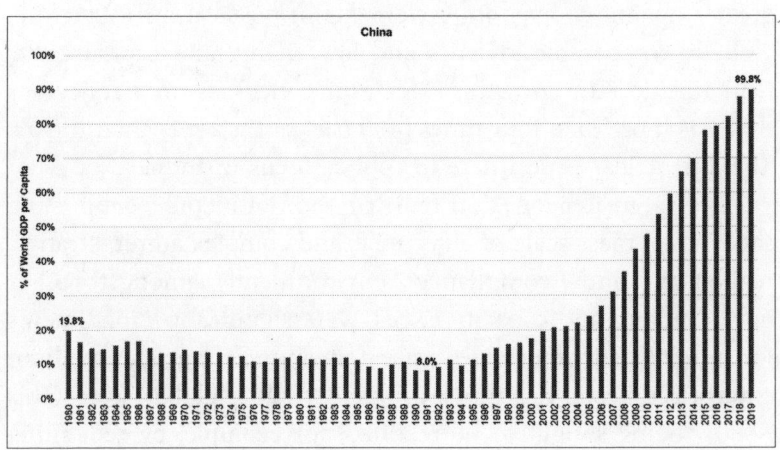

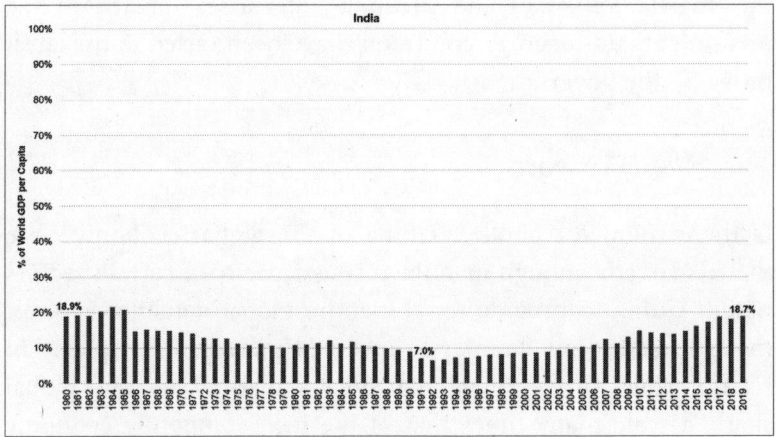

Source: World Bank

declined from being over 20 per cent of global per capita GDP in the early 1960s to less than 7 per cent in the early 1990s.

The inability to take sufficient advantage of external demand to build domestic competitiveness is evident in the hard reality that in comparison China's per capita income, which was similar to India's at 7–8 per cent in the early 1990s, increased to almost 90 per cent of the global average per capita income in 2019, compared to ours reaching only 19 per cent as pointed out. With greater openness, huge improvements in physical infrastructure, globally comparable logistics and low energy and capital costs, China achieved a growth in per capita incomes on a trajectory that was more than four times (400 per cent) steeper than India's. There is a clear lesson here for policy focus in India.

India's greater focus on redistribution of income, supporting sub-critical mass scale of enterprise, and complex administrative, regulatory and compliance environment, amongst other infrastructure and capacity issues, were significant impediments for Indian small enterprises scaling up and for large and medium enterprises becoming more competitive at a global scale. This is now being sought to be rectified, for example, by redefining the criteria for small and medium enterprises for whom the investment and turnover conditions have been raised in the latest move by the government.

The Way Forward

Is there room for another China in the global economy once there is already enough manufacturing capacity in certain sectors within China to provide for the entire global demand? Does it make sense for any country to invest in incremental capacity in sectors where China already has greater than 50 per cent global share, a scale many times that of the next competing economy (whether in the Organisation for Economic Co-operation and

Development [OECD] or the emerging group of countries)? With China now enjoying tremendous relative economies of scale, a much better developed ecosystem, and most importantly with its largest enterprises willing to compete at prices with low single-digit operating margins, and well below the lowest cost of production of the next most competitive economy, will anyone have the ability to compete? It will take tremendous effort to wrest some of the monopoly-like shares in world markets, across a large number of sectors, from China. However, the changing perception of global investors about the acute country risk in concentrating production capacities in one country and the need for diversification across different geographies presents India with an opportunity that must be seized to spur and sustain growth, going forward.

But clearly, the world is very different now as compared to at the turn of the century when China had a similar relative per capita GDP to the world average as India's today (19 per cent). China benefited from multiple tailwinds, including rising trade to global GDP ratios, improving demographics, lower debt to GDP ratio, etc. These are no longer available. Nonetheless, there are still many factors that support a strong case for India's faster relative ascendancy in the global economy—a demographic boom still ahead of us; among the lowest levels of private debt within large economies; the largest, broadest and deepest labour market in the world at low wages with low price elasticity; a very competitive stock market with bond markets improving rapidly; and the fifth largest GDP in the world to provide domestic demand to reach a competitive global scale. How can India ensure that it capitalizes on these massive opportunities and potential sources of strength?

Our answer is to use the present opportunity to ramp up the construction of physical infrastructure, thereby improving logistics and providing energy and capital inputs at globally comparable rates to our industry, which should be encouraged to target global competitive positions and shares.

Many established and well-meaning economists are asking for additional fiscal stimulus at this time. Among the most popular is the call for direct cash transfers (DCTs) to those most impacted, and if it is not easily possible to identify them, then to those at the bottom of the pyramid. The call for stimulus in the form of DCT is generally based on the assumption that more money in the bank accounts of the bottom 50–75 per cent of society will drive greater consumption and hence, higher capacity utilization for enterprises. The issue, however, is how much demand would it stimulate, for how long or how sustainably, and where will we find ourselves after the stimulus has worked its way through the economy?

Such a stimulus is likely to have a lower impact on encouraging incremental demand and consumption now than in other circumstances due to massive uncertainty engendered by the COVID-19 pandemic. This uncertainty affects both consumers and producers. It is evident in a continuing sequential rise in bank deposits. This, despite very low interest rates, including a continued 27-plus per cent year-on-year growth in balances in Jan Dhan bank accounts until August 2020, and despite the reality that these accounts belong to the lowest economic strata, which have already benefited from prior DCT under the PM Garib Kalyan Yojana.

In the face of such unprecedented uncertainty, consumer propensity to save has clearly not allowed the expected rise in consumption to materialize. Even for a fairly sizeable cash transfer, the increase in consumption is unlikely to increase capacity utilization of Indian industry from prevailing levels to higher than 80 per cent, which is normally the trigger for a new capital investment cycle. The short point is that money from this direct cash transfer for stimulating consumption would have run through the economy, providing temporary respite. However, this would have happened without leaving behind any improved competitive position, other than perhaps slightly better private balance sheets than otherwise, while leaving the government with a substantially higher debt load and less fiscal space going forward.

So, would it not be better to focus the stimulus on improving the competitive strength of India's enterprises, while enhancing ease of living and boosting employment, much more than just briefly stimulating overall consumption demand for the existing capacity?

A key recurring theme in India has been spreading meagre resources across too many fronts. Most initiatives don't deliver to their potential due to suboptimal funding and lack of focus to help them attain critical mass in terms of momentum. Fewer programmes with greater focus and resources will have substantially better overall results for the economy. In fact, consolidating and streamlining government programmes has been a key focus of the current government to make them more effective and increase the bang for buck of government spending. Also, a better, more rational sequencing of investments can greatly increase return on investment. For example, it would not make sense to build new factories before road access, energy and water are available in sufficient quantity and quality, and reliably, to the new site.

Therefore, we propose that an additional fiscal stimulus, regardless of size, should be focused primarily on driving better competitiveness for Indian enterprises and creating the greatest employment for the investment over the next six to 24 months. This would not just drive greater utilization of current capacity but also start the addition of new capacity as India becomes a more attractive destination for global production. The efficiencies and reduction in costs of goods and services will surely make

India more competitive in global markets. These will also create a consumer surplus domestically, which will result in greater savings and consumption by citizens, as well as improve the investment rate in the Indian economy. Policy measures to boost the economy should focus on improving the competitiveness of those segments of the Indian economy that have very high employment elasticity. These sectors are easily identifiable.

How do we achieve greater competitiveness and try and increase our share in global trade and global markets? We should accelerate approval of projects for the improvement of infrastructure, especially logistics, people transport, hospitality, power and communications, with a preference for PPP. The government should cede economic space with the privatization of public enterprises; ensuring the continuing transformation of the financial architecture of the country for better quality underwriting and better availability of risk capital; an optimal mix of banks, NBFCs and bonds to meet the credit needs of the economy; and making sure that insurance and pension penetration within the country rises faster. Collectively these measures could serve to accelerate India's GDP growth by 5 per cent annually from business as usual, with an annual increase in private credit to GDP by about 3–5 per cent for the next couple of decades.

Further improvement to competitiveness and near-term employment can come from a significant upgrade of our urban space and building stock, both in the redevelopment of poorly utilized, existing urban and rural settlements as well as new construction built to raise the standards of urban design and building as per the latest planning and construction norms. India's urban road networks require conduits for services (electricity, communications, water and sewage) to prevent frequent disruption and the incessant digging up of roads. The construction industry's employment elasticity of over 5 times the general economy could provide tremendous boost to employment and confidence. PPP has tremendous potential here with the government's participation through the provision of land and regulatory approvals, drawing in private capital and developers. This is the road to achieve sustained and rapid growth and convert the COVID-19-induced contingency into an opportunity for ramping up India's share in global FDI as also in world trade flows of goods and services.

Stimulating the direct consumption demand when our enterprises are not sufficiently competitive would be an inefficient prioritization of scarce resources. If successful in raising consumption levels, it would boost imports more than exports and also not trigger a fresh, virtuous cycle of investment. Focusing first on streamlining impediments to make Indian enterprises more competitive, which would, in turn, boost employment within three to six months and subsequently increase incremental demand for goods and services, would be a more optimal sequence of resource allocation. It would provide a far more sustainable recovery in a still uncertain global economic growth scenario that could remain sluggish for years.

Conclusion

There is an opportunity for India to build the latest and a globally comparable infrastructure, with the most competitive inputs in terms of quality and price for its enterprises, which will then have the opportunity to attain global scale and competitiveness. In a world of sluggish demand with systemic overcapacity and redundancies, amidst intensifying global competition and increasing protectionism with rising geopolitical stresses, Indian enterprises will see tremendous improvement in competitiveness at a time when it will count the most. India's economy could resume and sustain double-digit growth for the next three decades. This alone will suffice to meet the exploding aspirations of our young population. Let our response to COVID-19 put the Indian economy on a higher and more sustainable growth trajectory, thereby converting this crisis into an opportunity.

◆

Rajiv Kumar is the vice chairman, NITI Aayog, and chancellor, Gokhale Institute of Politics and Economics, Pune. He has been an economic advisor in the ministries of industry and finance.

Ajit Pai is distinguished expert, NITI Aayog, where he heads Economics and Finance and oversees Public Disinvestment. He is consultant to the vice chairperson of NITI Aayog. He was also the managing director at Thomas Weisel Partners and at Stifel Financial.

PANDEMIC AND THE DOLLAR: TOWARDS A CREDIBLE INDIAN RESPONSE

V. Anantha-Nageswaran

America Buries Volcker and Puts Dollar at Risk

On 27 August 2020, Jerome Powell, the chairman of the Federal Reserve Board in the US, unveiled a new monetary policy strategy for the institution he heads. The new framework would see the Federal Reserve tolerate a higher inflation rate while allowing the unemployment level to keep falling. Interest rates would stay low for longer. In other words, real interest rate would be negative for a long time. This is a 180-degree turnaround from the policy of Paul Volcker in the 1980s, which saw real interest rates in the US spike. This sent the US dollar soaring in the 1980s and cemented its dominance in the post-Bretton Woods world. Therefore, it is logical that this new framework would see the opposite effect on the dollar in the months and years ahead.

Inflation targeting began to be adopted as a mandate by the central bank in the 1980s because of the following factors: The experience of high inflation in the 1970s; the need to bring down long-term interest rates as economic growth had stalled after the post-World War II, and reconstruction-led economic growth had run its course; to constrain the power of elected representatives and to vest more powers with 'disinterested' (and, therefore, democratically unaccountable) elites and experts; and, finally, but most importantly, to restore the balance of power to capital, away from labour. Since then, the balance of power has stayed with capital.

In the developed world, inflation hasn't remained dormant for so long because central banks were successful in taming it. Volcker brought it down in the US in the 1980s but at the cost of two recessions. Afterwards, expanding global trade, the decline in crude oil price and the advent of e-commerce pitched in. Above all, the balance between capital and labour shifted in favour of capital. Globalization—outsourcing of jobs and offshoring of manufacturing—weakened workers' bargaining power, brought wages down and hence, operating costs remained lower. Profit margins could expand without end-user prices having to rise too much.

Thus, independent central banks targeting inflation did not tame inflation, but the erosion of labour power and the consequent moderation in wages did. Central banks had nothing to do with it. If central banks were responsible for lowering the inflation rate, they should have been able to push it up higher. Since the turn of the millennium, first in Japan, and since 2008 in other developed economies, central banks have tried valiantly to generate inflation but in vain.

In response to the COVID pandemic that caught the world unawares in February 2020, many developed countries have raised fiscal spending substantially and issued copious guarantees to the public to stave off unemployment. Public debt, already high, has climbed even higher. Developed countries need higher inflation to whittle down the real value of debt and other obligations that they owe to their people.

For inflation to raise its head, labour should acquire pricing power. It is highly likely that in the absence of rising labour power, Chairman Powell will fail in his mission to push up the inflation rate in the US. However, he may succeed more than he wishes to in undermining global trust and faith in the US dollar because his new policy framework comes at a time when the world is watching political and social developments in the US with rising alarm.

The US appears more divided than it has been at any time since the Civil War. It faced one of the most bitterly contested presidential elections on 3 November 2020, whose outcome is equally contested, if not more. Jack Goldstone and Peter Turchin wrote[18] that 'almost any election scenario this fall is likely to lead to popular protests on a scale we have not seen this century.' Therefore, political uncertainty and turmoil would compound the long-term uncertainty for the 'store of value' function of the US dollar that the new monetary policy framework has generated.

There is a possibility that the turmoil could mark the beginning of the end of the US dollar's reign as the dominant global reserve currency, especially if other rival nations sense an opportunity to begin the process of dismantling the dollar empire. Of course, global reserve currency status is not lost in a period of weeks or months, particularly since no other currency appears better placed than the US dollar to play that role now. In the meantime, the world may have to brace itself for a secular decline in the value of the dollar.

Bretton Woods Standard Ended in 1973

Developed nations ended fixed exchange rates when the successful post-World War II Bretton Woods system was abandoned in the 1970s. The US began to fret about the economic success of its World War enemies—Japan and Germany—although it had

---

[18]Jack A. Goldstone and Peter Turchin. (2020, September 10). 'Welcome to the Turbulent Twenties'. Accessed on https://www.noemamag.com/welcome-to-the-turbulenttwenties/

played a big role in their economic revival. It worried about losing competitive edge to them. In order to achieve competitiveness, it took a short cut. It decided to follow accommodative monetary policy and allow inflation to rise. Real rates in America began to decline from the mid-1960s onwards. Around the same time, America began to get deeply enmeshed in the Vietnam War. Fiscal deficit began to widen. Inflation picked up even further. In real terms, the dollar went nowhere in the 1960s. But, European nations began to demand gold from America in return for the overvalued dollar that they wanted to get rid of. The recession in the 1970s accelerated the decline of the dollar. President Richard Nixon took a unilateral decision to suspend the dollar-gold convertibility in 1971. Attempts made to stitch it back did not succeed. Exchange rates began to float in 1973.

Chart 1

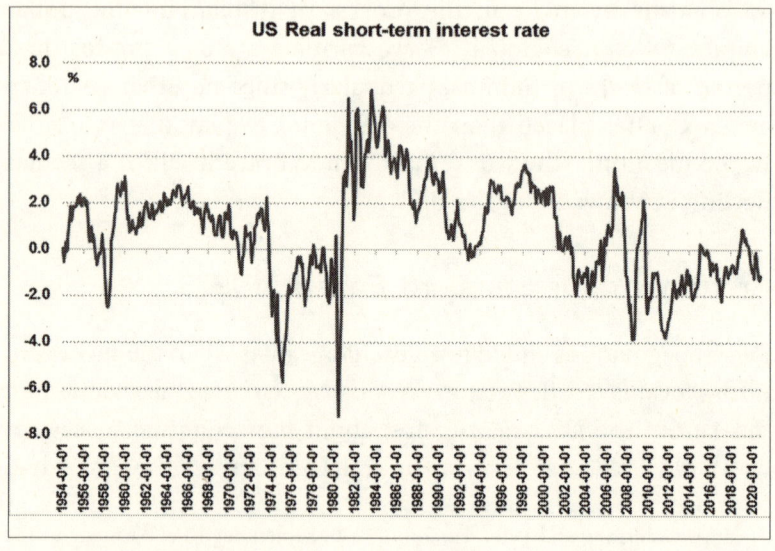

Source: Federal Reserve Bank of St. Louis Database

But, Dollar Standard Persisted

In the developing world, most countries pegged their currencies to the US dollar for it helped signal their anti-inflation credibility to the market. But, fixed exchange rates frequently led to surge in capital inflows, overheating and real exchange rate appreciation, as inflation rates spiked from time to time despite the commitment to low inflation. Or, overheating manifested itself in trade and CADs that needed funding. Emerging economies found themselves at the mercy of international financial institutions or international capital markets, which injured national pride. This played out vividly during the Asian crisis in 1997–98.

Therefore, very few emerging nations maintain a *de jure* peg to the hard currencies. Most countries have floated their exchange rates. However, they do wish to maintain a stable exchange rate, particularly versus the US dollar. Most of them still rely on the final demand from the American consumer to grow their economies. In other words, although the Bretton Woods system of fixed exchange rates was dismantled in the 1970s, there is a *de facto* fixed exchange rate regime with the US dollar as the anchor currency.

This synchronizes global economic cycles, and holds to this day. When the US lowers interest rates and maintains an accommodative monetary policy stance to rejuvenate the economy and sustain an economic expansion, other countries follow suit lest their currencies appreciate too much against the US dollar. But, their currencies appreciate nonetheless as a weak dollar spurs global risk appetite and leads to capital flowing into emerging economies seeking higher returns. Borrowers from emerging economies yield to the temptation to borrow in cheaper dollars and run up external debt. Usually, an abundance of capital leads to bad investment decisions by firms.

When the US monetary policy cycle starts to become more restrictive because, let us say, inflation picks up, or the US wants to slow down the economy, risk appetite weakens and the cycle reverses. Capital flows back into America. Emerging currencies depreciate. Their central banks, now afraid of the knock-on effects on their dollar borrowings (this is what happened in Asia in 1997–98), raise interest rates to prevent excessive currency weakness. So, their economies too slow down. This is how economic cycles around the world are synchronized. This also leads to synchronicity in capital markets—fixed income and stock markets. As a result, in reality, although there are 195 countries in the world, there has been a single economy (the US), one market (American stock and fixed income markets), one currency (US dollar) and one monetary policy (Federal Reserve) all these years.

2008: A Turning Point in the Dollar Standard

Dollar dominance had begun to change after the global financial crisis of 2008, though only gradually. In 2013, although the Federal Reserve did not raise interest rates, it threatened to slow down its purchase of US assets. That is, it threatened to reduce the quantum of the infusion of dollars into the economy. That was enough to send emerging market currencies tumbling. The Indian rupee was one of them. However, stability returned in 2014. When the Federal Reserve began to raise interest rates steadily in 2017–18, emerging market currencies did not come under strain, or did so only mildly.

Further, the US's economic growth rates had moderated post-crisis and despite record low interest rates and plenty of dollar liquidity, the country experienced one of the weakest economic recoveries since World War II, after the 2008 crisis. That was the main reason why global trade growth began to slow down after the 2008 crisis once the initial hopes of a rapid recovery to the pre-2008 normal faded. Subsequently, due to rising labour costs in China and concerns over the imbalances that globalization and liberalized trade had caused both domestically and globally, the US began to retreat from its commitments to a liberal trade regime, especially after Donald Trump became the 45th president of the country.

In other words, the policy of growing the economy by selling to the American consumer was no longer feasible. Emerging economies had to find other ways to grow. They have not. That is why economic growth rates in emerging markets have slowed sharply across the board. Those who are looking for answers specific to each country—such as demonetization, introduction of the GST, intrusive tax regimes, etc., as in the case of India, for instance—should pay closer to attention to common factors that have undermined economic growth in emerging economies.

TABLE 1
Real GDP Growth Rates for Emerging Economies

Country	2010	2011	2012	2013	2014	2015	2016	2017	2018	2019	2020	2021	Estimates Start After
Brazil	7.53	3.97	1.92	3.01	0.50	-3.55	-3.28	1.32	1.32	1.14	-5.80	2.83	2019
China	10.56	9.50	7.90	7.80	7.30	6.90	6.85	6.95	6.75	6.11	1.85	8.24	2019
India	10.26	6.64	5.46	6.39	7.41	8.00	8.26	7.04	6.12	4.18	-10.29	8.80	2019
Indonesia	6.38	6.17	6.03	5.56	5.01	4.88	5.03	5.07	5.17	5.03	-1.50	6.11	2019
Malaysia	7.53	5.29	5.47	4.69	6.01	5.01	4.45	5.81	4.77	4.30	-6.00	7.80	2019
Mexico	5.12	3.66	3.64	1.35	2.85	3.29	2.63	2.11	2.20	-0.30	-8.95	3.53	2019
Russia	4.50	5.07	4.02	1.76	0.74	-1.97	0.19	1.83	2.54	1.34	-4.12	2.82	2019
South Africa	3.04	3.28	2.21	2.49	1.85	1.19	0.40	1.42	0.79	0.15	-8.00	3.00	2019
Turkey	8.43	11.20	4.79	8.49	4.94	6.08	3.32	7.50	2.96	0.92	-4.99	5.00	2019

International Monetary Fund, World Economic Outlook Database, April 2020 (updated with June 2020 WEO updated, with revised growth estimates for 2020 and for 2021)

Source: IMF WEO Databases

So, to quickly summarize the developments so far, after World War II ended, the world agreed on a new monetary regime in which all currencies were pegged to the dollar and the dollar was pegged to gold, with the US offering convertibility between the US dollar and gold. It stopped working when the US wanted a shortcut out of eroding competitiveness. The era of floating exchange rates dawned in 1973. But, the world wanted stable exchange rates, emerging economies in particular. Countries behaved as though they were on a dollar standard, effectively sacrificing monetary policy autonomy and tying it to the Federal Reserve.

Post-2008, the arrangement began to fray as the Federal Reserve became unconventional and unilateral. It also became less effective as the American economy struggled to grow and was no longer the buyer of first and last resort for exporting nations. Furthermore, it walked out of trade agreements, tightened the screws on China and shut its face on globalization. In this milieu, two major developments have taken place.

The Pandemic Hastens the Arrival of the Post-Post-Bretton Woods Era

One is that the COVID pandemic struck in March. The world has not been able to satisfy itself thoroughly that it was natural. Further, to prevent the spread of the virus, countries chose to lock themselves down. The virus is still around and countries are still coping and adjusting to the new reality. Supply chain safety has now replaced supply chain sufficiency. Japan is incentivizing its companies to shift production out of China back to Japan and to a few other countries. Rising unemployment has forced many countries to tighten curbs on immigrant labour (e.g., Singapore) as the public clamours for jobs for locals. Therefore, reliance on export-led growth has taken a bigger knock than it took after the 2008 crisis and after Trump's foreign trade unilateralism.

The second development is the 180-degree turn in monetary policy that the US has taken. This is not a cyclical phenomenon.

It marks a break from the post-Bretton Woods era when the US still anchored the global monetary and currency regime, although increasingly imperfectly and unilaterally. Its unilateralism, which began in the late 1960s, ended the Bretton Woods arrangement. Its unilateralism is now going to upend the post-Bretton Woods arrangement, wherein emerging economies were operating on a *de facto* dollar standard as I had written earlier.

The attempt is to generate inflation and keep real interest rates as low as they were in the 1970s. What would it achieve? It would help the developed world whittle down the debt. Government obligations—real and contingent—have gone up steadily in the last 40 years. But, in the last 12 years, the rate of growth has picked up momentum. The ratio of public debt to GDP went up due to the rescues mounted to save the global financial system. Data from the Bank for International Settlements shows that the gross public debt-to-GDP ratio was 71 per cent at the end of 2007. By the end of 2011, it had risen to 100.4 per cent. It rose further to 114.6 per cent by mid-2016. It had begun to decline slowly but the pandemic has halted and reversed the descent. Debt ratios are set to rise very sharply. In its June 2020 update to the WEO, the IMF projects that the debt ratio for advanced nations would jump to 131.2 per cent of GDP from 105.2 per cent in 2019, and for the advanced G20 nations, it would jump to 141.4 per cent from 113.2 per cent. For both the groups, it worsens further into 2021 as well.

So, left with a crushing debt burden, not to mention social security and pension obligations that represent promises made in good times and are contingent liabilities, developed countries are looking for an encore of the 1970s when the inflation rate was in double digits, real interest rates were persistently negative and debt ratios plunged. See the charts below for the success achieved in reducing the debt ratios in the UK and in the US. This is the unstated objective now for the decade of the 2020s.

Chart 2

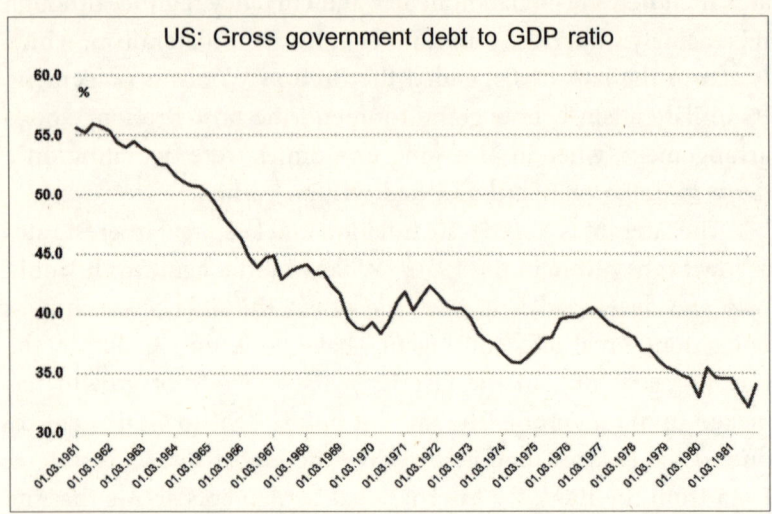

Source: 'Credit to the Non-Financial Sector', Bank for International Settlements (June 2020 version)

Chart 3

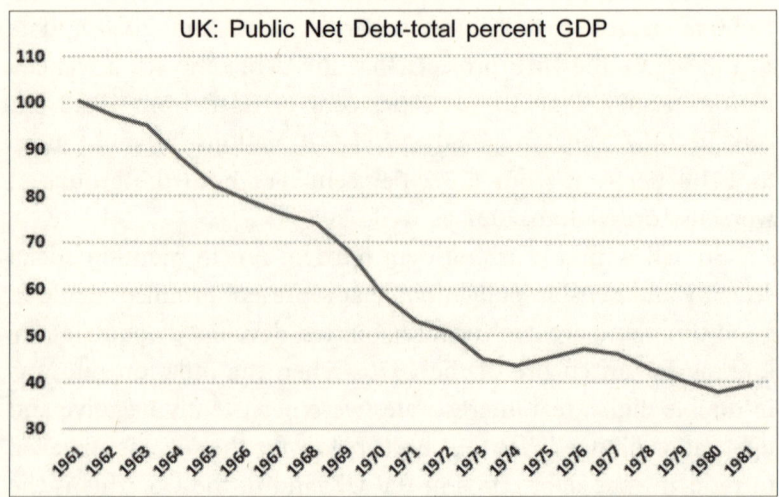

Source: https://www.ukpublicspending.co.uk/uk_national_debt_analysis

Whether central banks achieve this goal or not is an altogether different question. Much depends on whether wages rise. Without the support from wage growth, it may be harder to generate inflation. Workers' preference for real wage growth, as they see through the attempt of central banks to generate inflation, will erode profit share and end the outsized gains to capital of the last three decades. That sets the stage for social conflicts. Therefore, whether or not the Federal Reserve and other central banks (in the UK, Europe and Japan) succeed in generating inflation, they may succeed in debasing their currencies as the risk of holding them rises in the coming years. This is unlikely to be a transient phenomenon. It may culminate in the need for and the formulation of another global monetary regime. But, the path from here to there will be rough, and developing nations have to abandon their familiar routine of the last 20 years.

Emerging economies have to make major policy choices of their own, in response to all these developments, amidst extreme economic uncertainty. They have to figure out an economic growth strategy and an exchange rate management strategy, which are not dependent on the West. They cannot take their cues from them and follow their lead. They have to get down to the hard work of generating domestic production and domestic growth. Postponing hard choices and hiding behind high economic growth are no longer feasible. Growth cannot paper over cracks and present a veneer of success. That won't come by easily. Emerging economies have to make major policy choices of their own, in response to all these developments, amidst extreme economic uncertainty.

India, in particular, has been battling a fragile banking system for the last several years. Both banks and their corporate clients have been bogged down by too much debt, which become unpayable. India's economic growth rate had slowed sharply in the last few years. While it is true that India is not an outlier in this regard, India's population size and its demographics (higher proportion of youth) make the growth shortfall a serious problem in its own right.

What Should India Do?

Until now, India has been behaving like other developing economies. It has resisted currency strength by buying dollars and holding down the value of the rupee. Foreign exchange reserves held by the RBI, as of 4 September 2020, were a little under $500 billion. Over the last one year, it has increased by $101 billion. If the US dollar goes into a sustained free fall, continuing with this strategy will present India with rising costs and other challenges.

The RBI will be required to keep buying dollars to prevent the rupee from appreciating and to avoid recognizing losses on the purchase of dollars in the last two years. It is a road to nowhere. It might end up being a case of the tiger chasing its tail. It will never succeed. That would erode revaluation reserves. Together with a non-existent return on foreign currency assets, holding foreign exchange reserves might become an exorbitant burden rather than a sign of strength as in the past. It is a paradigm shift and we may have to abandon old response patterns because the reality has changed.

If the RBI keeps intervening, it would build up reserves and enable domestic credit to flow to zombie assets or stock market speculation or both. But, the RBI would have to actively and continuously buy foreign currency because not doing so will mean incurring and realizing losses on existing foreign currency assets. It is a treadmill, and the equivalent of retail investors averaging down. They have no choice if the Federal Reserve is going to let the dollar sink.

The other option is to let the market determine the level of the rupee without distorting it with interventions. It has many advantages. For one, it will be cleaner. The RBI will not have to accumulate foreign assets that yield nothing and that keep losing value. In the process, it has also had to intervene to lessen the impact of its dollar purchase on domestic money supply. One intervention begets another. Two, it will force Indian businesses to become productive and efficient. It takes time, no doubt. But there is no history of countries depreciating their currencies on the way to prosperity. Japan, Switzerland and Germany are three countries that achieved trade competitiveness despite the strength of their currencies. Some would say because of it.

In general, contrary to popular perception and the claims of an export lobby, a cheap currency is no panacea for exports. Income effects dominate the price effect. In the new millennium, India's non-oil exports surged despite the Indian rupee strengthening in value. To be sure, India's imports surged too. But, it would be a mistake to attribute it solely to the strength of the currency, making imports cheaper and hence attractive. India's economic growth took off and that sucked in imports. Once again, it was the case of income effect at work.

Chart 4

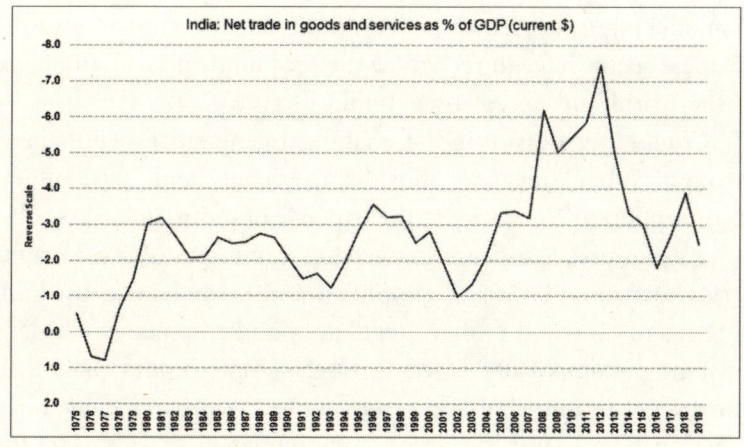

Source: World Bank Metadata

Embrace Strong Currency and Structural Reforms

However, a strong currency could induce complacency among businesses, tempting them to borrow in foreign currencies. The risk of it creating balance sheet stress for such borrowers in the event of a sudden crash in the rupee is substantial. For an Indian financial system that is fragile, such a risk might be too big to bear. Repaying foreign currency loans requires export earnings, which might be hard to come by, given weak global growth and rising preference for domestic manufacturing in many countries. Indeed, a strong currency could potentially undermine India's thrust on self-reliance, as imports appear cheaper with a strong domestic currency.

India faces difficult choices here. Sticking to business as usual will be increasingly difficult and costlier whereas currency strength is a powerful weapon that can hurt if not handled properly. What should the Indian government and central bank do?

As mentioned earlier, in the long-run, depreciating currencies is a sign of economic underperformance and not strength. Therefore, preparing and placing the country in a position to reap the benefits of a strong currency is likely more rewarding than sticking to current practices. Both the government and the business sector have to recognize the profound shifts taking place in the world and accept their implications.

Competitiveness of Indian manufacturing must be enhanced through other means. Subsidizing retail and agricultural consumption of electricity at the expense of industrial users must be re-examined. Land-use conversion from agriculture to non-agriculture must be eased, simplified and made less costly, both in terms of time and money. Regulatory and compliance burdens must be systematically eased through a time-bound plan with transparent monitoring and reporting to the public. States must come on board, and the union government must kick-start the process with a summit of chief ministers.

Despite recent re-classification of MSMEs, the new thresholds do not go far enough in incentivizing their growth. They remain growth-unfriendly. They need to be revisited. Payments to MSMEs for goods sold and services rendered must happen automatically. Both government and private sector buyers are guilty. GST invoices and the government's e-procurement must be automatically linked to the Trade Receivables System. It is technologically feasible but behavioural feasibility must be mandated with severe penalties for non-compliance.

If these changes happen, then India can have the best of both worlds: a strong currency and strong economic fundamentals, with the former reflecting the latter. However, 'business as usual' with the central bank resisting rupee appreciation in a futile bid will succeed only in weakening the economy in multiple ways.

The fallout of the pandemic is upending familiar behaviour patterns and policy responses. The sooner we recognize them, the stronger we would emerge. I am not even sure that there is another option.

◆

V. Anantha-Nageswaran is a member of the PMEAC. He has worked with several international financial institutions. His co-authored books include *Economics of Derivatives* (2015), *Derivatives* (2017) and *The Rise of Finance: Causes, Consequences and Cures* (2020), all published by Cambridge University Press, UK.

POLICY OPTIONS FOR POST-COVID GROWTH

Arvind Virmani

The Indian economy is presently (July–December 2020) going through the transition from lockdown to normalization. Starting around 22 March 2020, the Government of India imposed the most comprehensive lockdown in the world. Only essential goods and services, constituting an estimated 40 per cent of GDP and 55 per cent of employment, were exempt from the lockdown. From mid-May the government started lifting the lockdown gradually and by end-June, it was largely eliminated at the central level.

The lockdown of 60 per cent of the economy for six weeks in April–June 2020 was enough to reduce the GDP for Q1 (April–June) of 2020–21 by 25 per cent below the GDP in April–June 2019. The GDP and the Index of Industrial Production (IIP) data confirm that the exempt sectors were the least affected by the lockdown. The ratio of Q1 GDP in FY21 to that in FY20 from agriculture and allied services was 13, and electricity, gas, water and other utilities at 0.93. Even mixed sectors with some lockdown component, such as financial, real estate and business services, had a ratio of 0.93, and that of exempt sectors with some lockdown component, such as public administration and other services (which include health, education and non-governmental organizations [NGOs]), was at 0.90.

A similar confirmation is obtained within the manufacturing

sector, measured by the ratio of IIP in April–May 2020 over 2019. For food products, the ratios were 0.75 and 1.3; for pharmaceutical and medicinal products, 0.46 and 12; for wood and related products, 0.87 and 1.4; and for refined petroleum products, 0.72 and 0.76. Some sectors, such as aerated beverages, hygiene-related chemical products, such as different types of packaging for essential goods, where the exemption was unclear, and products like tobacco and liquor, which were initially locked down, recovered quickly as soon as it became clear that they were part of the exemption.

This part of the economy, contributing 40 per cent to total GDP and 55 per cent to total employment, was functioning normally, with demand equal to supply, and wages, employment and profits close to normal. It also had a positive saving rate as its demand for goods and services produced by the rest of the economy could not be met because of complete or partial lockdown.

The rest of the economy, constituting 60 per cent of GDP and 45 per cent of employment, was subject to lockdown. In terms of broad GDP sectors, this consisted of manufacturing, mining and quarrying, and construction, and a large part of trade, hotels and transport; real estate, housing and business services; and other services. The ratio of Q1 GDP in FY21 to that in FY20 from construction was 0.5; for manufacturing, 0.61; and for mining, 0.77. The ratio for trade, hotels, transport, communication and broadcasting, at 0.53, was close to the locked-down construction sector, as the non-exempt communication and broadcasting sub-sectors constituted only a small part of the overall sector, and even exempt parts of the trade and transport sector serving essential commodities were disrupted by random bureaucratic actions at the state and local levels. The corresponding ratios (FY21:FY20) for average Q1 IIP for mining and manufacturing, at 0.78 and 0.59, are remarkably close to the GDP ratios. We can therefore use the IIP sub-aggregates to see the effect on individual industries.

The lockdown was complete and comprehensive in the capital goods and consumer goods sectors, with the ratio of April 2020 IIP to April 2019 IIP falling to zero. The industries that completely shut down in April were motor vehicles and other transport equipment, tobacco products, leather products, furniture, apparel and textiles, fabricated metal products, electrical equipment, computer and electrical products, and machinery and equipment. With the partial lifting of the lockdown in May, recovery was most rapid for apparel, furniture, metal products, leather products and tobacco products. In June, the worst affected capital goods and consumer goods sectors were textiles (0.46), motor vehicles (0.52) and other transport equipment (0.5), apparel (0.6), paper products (0.6), electrical equipment (0.62) and metal products (0.65).

This part of the economy contributing 60 per cent to total GDP and 45 per cent to total employment was therefore shut down during April 2020, with both supply and the effective demand equal to zero. There was also no scope for use of a conventional fiscal policy stimulus to raise aggregate demand, which would have had zero effect on demand. With lockdown, wages, employment and profits all became zero. Every participant of this part of the economy had to use his/her accumulated savings to buy essential goods and services, resulting in negative savings rate.

Those who did not have any savings to fall back on or could not get family loans to survive were completely dependent on governments, NGOs and personal charity from their former employers for survival. Further, with zero or negative profits because of legally committed payments or arbitrary state government orders, there was a possibility of wholesale bankruptcy of firms heavily indebted in this part of the economy.

During the lockdown, the primary requirement from government (central and state) was to ensure against starvation and extreme deprivation of workers and the self-employed, as well as mass bankruptcies in the locked-down sectors constituting 60 per cent of GDP and 45 per cent of employment. The latter goal was shared with the RBI, which had to ensure that credit reached all those companies that were basically solvent but suffered from unprecedented liquidity problems arising from a government-ordained lockdown of their industry or services. The problem became less acute but continued during the phased lifting of the lockdown in May and June. It has persisted thereafter, with some states, towns and districts going for partial lockdowns and the fears aroused among workers, firms and consumers by the resurgence of the pandemic. The focus of the central and state governments, along with the RBI, therefore remained on minimizing the possibility of extreme deprivation and mass bankruptcy, during Q2 of FY21.

As state governments lifted the lockdown at a different pace in different areas and others reimposed lockdown after lifting it, logistic chains from the producer to the final consumer as well as among different producers were disrupted. This has raised logistic costs, fragmented supply chains and produced pockets of excess supply and excess demand in different goods in different geographical areas. This was predicted by the EGROW Foundation research paper[19] on the economics of the pandemic and the lockdown. The rise in logistic costs is reflected in the rise of the ratio of the CPI to wholesale price index for food products during Q1 of FY21 and further to its highest level in July 2020.

Given that India is a large federal country, with constitutional powers divided between the central government and the states, the lockdown and other restrictions have been differentially implemented, creating uncertainty in the minds of the public and

---

[19] Arvind Virmani. (2020, September). *Policy for Post-Lockdown Indian Economy*, EGROW Foundation, New Delhi.
Accessed at: https://egrowfoundation.org/research/policy-for-post-lockdown-indian-economy/

raising risk. One of the few available measures of uncertainty is the National Stock Exchange Volatilty Index. This shows a 3.5 times increase in uncertainty in March 2020 when the pandemic started in India and the government started imposing restrictions. It came down to 3 times in April when the lockdown was announced and 2 times in June when it was being lifted. By August 2020 it was down to 1.4 times its level in February 2020.

Among the sectors that were locked down, it's important to distinguish between those that have some contagion possibilities because of close personal interaction with strangers but were more affected by the lockdown (manufacturing, mining, construction, goods transport, storage, repair services), and those that are directly and heavily affected by the pandemic and fears of contagion and death. The latter has been defined in our research as 'contact services' in which consumption/purchase involves contact with many other consumers/buyers. These sectors are restaurants, hotels, public transport, wholesale and retail trade (except ecommerce) and other services such as hospitality, entertainment and tourism. There are genuine fears with respect to these sectors, which will continue for much longer.

To minimize contagion, the fears connected to it and to restore confidence, it's essential that all governments, employers, workers, self-employed, NGOs and consumers follow the following precautions that science has taught us so far about COVID-19. This is the only way to a sustained normalization of the economy:

1. *Hygiene* (sterilization) and frequent *handwashing*, particularly before touching your mouth, ears or nose.
2. Wear *masks* in the presence of others (non-family member and infected family member). A triple (or double) layer cotton mask, covering the nose and mouth, seems most appropriate for Indian weather conditions.
3. *Keep physical distance* if (a) in a closed area with non-

family members; (b) eating, drinking or speaking directly with someone; or (c) the other person is without a mask.
4. *Well-ventilated areas*, halls and rooms are safer than closed air-conditioned ones. Air-conditioned halls and rooms can be made as safe as well-ventilated ones by using ultraviolet purification of, or virus-quality filters for, recirculated air. Ultraviolet roof lights are being developed for cleaning room air but are not yet available.
5. *Crowded bars*, indoor parties and public bathrooms are dangerously prone to coronavirus spread. Older and vulnerable people should avoid them.
6. *Testing, tracing and quarantine* is a chain in which the quality depends on the weakest link. Home quarantine requires that all members of household follow the above precautions with respect to the quarantined member. Similar care is required in public quarantine facilities, clinics and hospitals to ensure that they do not themselves spread the coronavirus instead of containing it.

Based on our analysis of the exempt and lockdown sectors, it is possible to calculate the effect of lockdown on GDP. For arithmetic simplicity, assume that lockdown was fully operational for the first one and a half months of Q1 FY21 and completely lifted during the rest of Q1. The arithmetic then shows a (-)25 per cent decline (year on year) in Q1 2020–21 GDP. The actual decline was (-)23.5 per cent (year on year).

There is extremely limited data available for Q2 FY21. The Centre for Monitoring of Indian Economy's (CMIE) monthly unemployment rate (UR%) is useful for getting a preliminary picture of the current situation. The ratio of the UR% in 2020 to that in 2019 provides a useful indicator, like the IIP ratio used earlier. This ratio was 1.1 in February and 1.3 in March, indicating a 20 per cent higher pre-pandemic UR% because of the GDP growth slowdown in 2019–20. With the introduction of the lockdown, this UR% ratio shot up to 3.2 in April and 3.3 in May and dropped back to 1.4 in June after the lockdown started lifting. Surprisingly, it is down to 1 in July and August, indicating a normalization of employment in Q2 FY21.

There is a caveat: the labour force participation rate (LFPR) declined during the pandemic and remains 2 percentage points above the average of 2019–20. This is consistent with the fears of contagion and of contacting the pandemic when using public transport and working in a factory office or shop with many others present. CMIE data also indicates that the LFPR has declined the most among salaried employees, less among the casual labour and least among the self-employed. This is also consistent with the hypothesis that the better educated, wealthier individuals have the knowledge and the wealth to temporarily withdraw from the job market, while the pandemic rages. Finally, the CMIE data also shows that the greatest change in LFPR is in Haryana, a state bordering Delhi, which has among the highest number of COVID cases, and whose modern industries and services are located in Faridabad and other towns close to Delhi.

We define post-pandemic economic normalization as attaining a level for major economic indicators, such as GDP, IIP or UR%, equal to that prevailing in the corresponding period a year ago. The transition from lockdown to normalization is under way in Q2 and is likely to continue in Q3 FY21. It is critical to sustained recovery that the COVID precautions outlined earlier be strictly followed. During this transition period, fiscal–monetary coordination is critical. Monetary policy must maintain high liquidity, low and stable real interest rates in the market for all systemically significant instruments. All segments of the credit market must continue to be assured through government credit guarantees. Because of the fragmentation of supply chains and markets during the pandemic, a conventional aggregated fiscal stimulus will not be useful but could also stoke inflation in areas of excess demand, without stimulating demand in areas with excess supply. We need sector-specific fiscal stimulus directed at sectors with weak demand. The government also needs to put in place a number of structural policy reforms during the transition, which would be critical to restoring fast growth following normalization.

There are several economic trends that originated before the pandemic but have been enhanced by it. India is in a position to grab the opportunity with the joint effort of private business, governments and NGOs. These are:

1. Deglobalization of trade, FDI and the movement of people. Atmanirbhar Bharat and the greater acceptability of remote work are positives.
2. High-tech decoupling between the US and China provides greater opportunity for shifting value chains to India, given that many Fortune 500 companies already have research and development (R&D) centres here, and there is a large supply of educated labour. However, the provision of job skills needs to be strengthened immediately.
3. Export supply chain diversification from China was initiated by Trump's tariff war, but China's behaviour during the pandemic has strengthened these trends.
4. Digitization has progressed much faster in the developed countries than in India. The pandemic will accelerate the trend in India. There is an opportunity to innovate in e-governance, e-education/skilling, e-medicine/health, e-commerce and remote working.
5. Environment concerns will be heightened. We are well placed with our solar initiatives and can start with an electric vehicle policy.
6. Public health, nutrition and health education concerns

will take centre stage for some years. We can expand and deepen Swachh Bharat to overhaul the nation's sewage, solid waste collection, and processing and disposal systems from end to end.

Based on the above analysis, I would recommend the following policies:

1. Reform textiles import duties by replacing all specific duties with a uniform ad valorem tariff.
2. Integrate all GST rates on different textile raw materials, fibres, fabrics and garments into a single rate, which, in a broader GST simplification, should be 15 per cent. The diversity of rates on cotton and manmade/artificial fibres/fabrics has left us out of global textile supply chains and progressively lowered our ranking in textile and ready-made garment exports.
3. Reduce GST on commercial vehicles, consumer durables and capital goods, currently at 28 per cent, to 25 per cent, and those at 18 per cent, to 15 per cent.
4. Integrate all subsides into a DBT/DCT system. To ensure ease of living, DCTs should be delivered directly to all rural residents and migrants on their mobile phones, with the husband and wife (one or both of whom could be migrants), receiving their share separately and the share of minor children delivered to the mothers' cell phones. This will ensure that the bottom 40 per cent can be financially protected from any future disasters.
5. To promote the acquisition of skills to move labour from casual to regular work, amend the Apprenticeship Act to make it easy to impart practical job skills, without being subject to inflexible labour laws.
6. Previously planned infrastructure and housing projects must be revived and accelerated.

7. A 'strategic industry policy' should be formally approved and implemented through privatization, equity and land sale as per policy.
8. The three acts proposing simplification of labour laws are now before Parliament and should be passed after deleting clauses that reduce flexibility. While the fourth labour law is being formulated, the special economic zone (SEZ) law should be revised to introduce flexibility in retrenching workers made redundant by demand fluctuations.
9. Ease of doing business can be enhanced by reducing the number of regulations, eliminating criminal penalties and facilitating digital filling/filing of simplified forms followed by randomized post audits to ensure implementation of critical regulations relating to health, safety and environment. This can be included in the SEZ law amendment while the general simplification is devised.
10. Import substitution policy should be strictly restricted to the few countries that are known to have used asymmetric trade, FDI and technology policies, while a freer trade approach is adopted for all other countries. The supply chain resilience initiative, product-linked incentives and consumer goods tariffs should be on goods exported by such countries.
11. Reduce the differential, higher electricity price for industry as proposed in the amendment to the Electricity Act (2003). Set up common treatment centres for chemical plants to attract supply chains.
12. Rationalize and simplify GST by choosing one of the two options proposed by the author, with new rates effective from 1 April 2021. Rationalize and simplify the Direct Tax Code as per the 255-page law proposed in August 2009. These tax reforms are essential for Atmanirbhar Bharat as they will level the playing field for small and

medium enterprises to compete with companies [given the excellent corporate tax reform (2019)].

The Indian economy has been set back by a series of events, resulting in a FY20 GDP growth of 4.2 per cent and a projected FY21 growth of (-)5 per cent -/+ 2.5 per cent with downward bias. The pessimistic view is that GDP growth will be negative or zero even in FY22. A crisis of this magnitude is a terrible thing to waste. I am an optimist; in my view a growth take-off is possible in FY22, if we complete all pending reforms by end-March 2021.

◆

Arvind Virmani is currently chairman, Foundation for Economic Growth and Welfare, New Delhi. He was chief economic advisor, Government of India, and principal economic advisor, Planning Commission. He also served as an executive director on the board of the International Monetary Fund.

THE POLITICAL ECONOMY OF UNCERTAINTY

Sanjaya Baru

In a perceptive and early comment on the policy challenge posed by the COVID-19 pandemic, and more importantly, the sudden and comprehensive economic lockdown imposed, the chairman of the PMEAC, Bibek Debroy, reminded us of a key postulate we owe to economists Frank Knight and John Maynard Keynes: 'Risk has a known probability distribution. For uncertainty, the probability distribution is unknown. COVID-19 makes us confront uncertainty, not risk.'[20]

Writing a month after the nationwide lockdown was imposed, Debroy was drawing attention to the prevalent uncertainty about the nature and extent of the impact of the pandemic and the consequent public policy choices that needed to be made by the government. Given that both the pandemic, in its scope and character, and the draconian lockdown were unprecedented, the government was functioning in an environment of uncertainty, which its own actions had further accentuated. Knight's 1921 treatise on uncertainty and risk drew attention to the distinction between the two in economic decision-making, stating:

---

[20]Bibek Debroy. (2020, April 25). 'Risk, uncertainty and Covid-19: A Stark Choice'. *Financial Express*. Accessed at: https://www.financialexpress.com/opinion/risk-uncertainty-and-covid-19-a-stark-choice/1939070/

> Uncertainty must be taken in a sense radically distinct from the familiar notion of Risk, from which it has never been properly separated... The essential fact is that 'risk' means in some cases a quantity susceptible of measurement... It will appear that a measurable uncertainty, or 'risk' proper, as we shall use the term, is so far different from an unmeasurable one that is not in effect an uncertainty at all. We shall accordingly restrict the term 'uncertainty' to cases of the non-quantitative type.[21]

Over a decade later, and having lived through the Great Depression, Keynes offered a more policy-oriented view of uncertainty. In an essay in the *Quarterly Journal of Economics* explaining the essence of his path-breaking book, *The General Theory of Employment, Interest and Money* (1936), Keynes clearly distinguished between what we may term as a 'predictable uncertainty' and an 'unpredictable' one. To quote:

> I do not mean merely to distinguish between what is known for certain from what is only probable. The game of roulette is not subject, in this sense, to uncertainty.... The expectation of life is only slightly uncertain. Even the weather is only moderately uncertain. The sense in which I am using the term is that in which the prospect of a European war is uncertain, or...the rate of interest twenty years hence... About these matters there is no scientific basis on which to form any calculable probability whatever. We simply do not know.[22]

Combining the Knight–Keynes view of the role of uncertainty in economic decisions, with Keynes's profound observations on

---

[21] Frank H. Knight. (2006). *Risk, Uncertainty and Profit*. Dover Publications Inc, New York. (First edition published by Houghton Mifflin Company. Boston, 1921.) pp. 19–20

[22] John Maynard Keynes. (1937). 'The General Theory of Employment', *Quarterly Journal of Economics*, Vol. 51, Issue 2. p. 214

the role of expectations, one can appreciate the role of human response to events and policies in shaping economic outcomes. Where uncertainty about the future does not overwhelm human behaviour, expectations based on past and present experiences shape future outcomes. Risk is measurable and so are outcomes. However, when uncertainty grips individuals and societies, neither the past nor the present are reliable guides to the future.

Public policy and its effective and credible communication assume vital importance in dealing with the challenge of uncertainty. At the time when Debroy made the distinction between risk and uncertainty, neither medical doctors nor government officials could reasonably be expected to answer a wide range of questions posed by both the pandemic and the lockdown. Those who were brave enough to make forecasts and probabilistic statements succeeded in hitting media headlines, but most have been overtaken by events. There is still a lack of clarity on both the epidemiological possibilities and the economic consequences of the pandemic and the lockdown, respectively.

More worrying for the economy, there is still no clarity on the extent of damage inflicted by the virus and the lockdown on lives and livelihoods. Even if both these can be estimated, there is uncertainty about how various economic agents—consumers, investors, savers, the salaried and the self-employed—are likely to respond in years ahead, given the new uncertainties created by changing methods and habits of work, employment, spending and saving. While the Government of India's chief economic advisor bravely forecasts a V-shaped recovery for economic growth, many analysts foresee prolonged uncertainty thwarting that possibility.[23] The range of possibilities is becoming wider, with the growth

---

[23]Ruchi Bhatia. (2020, September). 'Worst is over, India experiencing a V-shaped recovery: CEA'. *The Economic Times*. Accessed at: https://economictimes.indiatimes.com/markets/expert-view/worst-is-over-india-experiencing-a-v-shaped-recovery-cea/articleshow/77864262.cms

recovery trajectory seen to follow K, L, U, V, W and Z shapes.[24] Simply articulating pessimistic or optimistic forecasts, like many anti- and pro-government economists are doing, can hardly help.[25] Credible and timely communication is key to effective policymaking even in normal times, and given COVID-19's uncertainty, one cannot overemphasize their importance.

◆

Economic policymakers in India have been used to managing a range of economic, political and external risks, as well as the uncertainty created by one-time disruptions ranging from a BoP crisis to an earthquake, tsunami, assassination of top leaders and even a limited war. Few, if any, have had the experience of dealing with prolonged uncertainty of the kind presented by an all-out war or a pandemic caused by a mutating virus. Analysts Scott Baker, Nicholas Bloom, Steven Davies and Stephen Terry have tried to measure 'COVID-induced economic uncertainty' and conclude that:

> The COVID-19 pandemic has triggered a massive spike in uncertainty. Major uncertainties surround almost every aspect: the infectiousness, prevalence, and lethality of the virus; the

---

[24]'7 ways India's economy could crawl out of Covid pit'. (2020, September). *Times of India*, New Delhi.

[25]See, for example, interventions in the media by Raghuram Rajan and Arvind Panagariya: Raghuram Rajan. (2020, September). 'GoI's plan to conserve resources for a future stimulus is self-defeating'. *The Economic Times*. Accessed at: https://economictimes.indiatimes.com/news/economy/policy/view-gois-plan-to-conserve-resources-for-a-future-stimulus-is-self-defeating/articleshow/77965769.cms

Arvind Panagariya. (2020, September). 'End of the World Isn't Nigh'. *The Economic Times*. Accessed at: https://economictimes.indiatimes.com/news/economy/policy/double-digit-slump-isnt-the-end-of-the-world-assures-arvind-panagariya/articleshow/78045135.cms

availability and deployment of antigen and antibody tests; the capacity of healthcare systems to meet an extraordinary challenge; how long it will take to develop and deploy safe, effective vaccines; the ultimate size of the mortality shock; the duration and effectiveness of social distancing, market lockdowns, and other mitigation and containment strategies; the near-term economic impact of the pandemic and policy responses; the speed of recovery as the pandemic recedes; whether 'temporary' government interventions and policies will persist; the extent to which pandemic-induced shifts in consumer spending patterns will persist; and the impact on business survival, new business formation, R&D, human capital investment, and other factors that affect productivity over the medium and long term.[26]

The authors have pioneered an Economic Policy Uncertainty Index (EPUI) that seeks to measure the incidence of uncertainty in an economy by gathering data from mainstream media in the 26 major economies that they monitor. In India, the EPUI team monitors seven major newspapers: *The Times of India*, *The Economic Times*, *The Indian Express*, *The Financial Express*, *Hindustan Times*, *The Hindu* and *The Statesman*. The index measures the frequency with which words like 'uncertainty' and 'economic policy' occur in these publications along with incidences of news coverage on fiscal, monetary and trade policies. The EPUI team finds a global spike in reporting on economic uncertainty from the early part of 2020. However, in the case of India, policy uncertainty is seen to be a recurring feature, albeit with a sharper spike since March 2020 (Table 1).

---

[26]Scott R. Baker, Nicholas Bloom, Steven J. Davis and Stephen J. Terry. (2020, April). 'Covid Induced Economic Uncertainty'. NBER Working Paper 26983. Accessed at: http://policyuncertainty.com/media/COVID-Induced%20 Economic%20Uncertainty.pdf

TABLE 1
India: Economic Policy Uncertainty Index

	2019	*2020*
January	64.7383	48.1354
February	50.1197	92.6491
March	40.4534	110984
April	60.4534	160.8216
May	83.6425	167.7502
June	72.8534	75.1469
July	70.4508	108.1987
August	81.6747	113834
September	105.5443	-
October	90.6638	-
November	50.3646	-
December	106355	-
Average	73829	109.4855

Source: Global EPUI (2020)

Consider the numbers. The Global EPUI increased from an annual average of 267 in calendar year 2019 to 320 in the first eight months of 2020 (January–August). For India, the average EPUI was 73.1 in 2019 and increased to 109.5 in January–August 2020.[27] Clearly, the spike in policy uncertainty in India in the post-COVID period is in step with global trends, but it was sharper than the spike in the global average. The kind of uncertainty gripping economic agents today is unprecedented. The uncertainty attached to economic phenomenon, such as demand for manufactured goods, investment in real estate, internal and international trade, travel and tourism, availability of migrant labour and so on, is even more unprecedented.

---

[27]Global EPUI 2020. Accessed at: http://policyuncertainty.com/global_monthly.html

Given this increased uncertainty, individual expectations would be suitably moderated, impacting macroeconomic outcomes. The economic consequence of heightened uncertainty has been noted in the RBI's annual report for 2019–20, which has drawn attention to the 'shock to consumption', to the fact that the 'precautionary savings instinct' has 'gripped businesses and households amidst heightened risk aversion' and to the 'evaporation' of the 'appetite for investment'. It concludes rightly so that 'behavioural restraints may prevent the normalisation of demand'.[28] The RBI's survey for July 2020 showed that consumer confidence had fallen to 'an all-time low, with a majority of respondents reporting pessimism relating to the general economic situation, employment, inflation and income.'[29] While respondents expected recovery in the year ahead and there was some optimism about improvements in rural consumption, the report noted that 'the appetite for investment is anaemic and in need of more reforms'. Going forward, the focus of public policy will have to be on altering the state of expectations and reducing uncertainty.

◆

One can possibly draw a parallel to the kind of uncertainty gripping economic agents as a consequence of COVID-19 and the lockdown with the experience of most European economies during World War II. A large number of industrial economies that were growing rapidly, contributing to rising consumption, trade, banking and financial services and so on, were suddenly caught in a devastating war that destroyed industrial capacity, disrupted the financial economy and services such as education and transportation. While COVID-19 has not destroyed industrial

---

[28]Reserve Bank of India (2020, August). *Annual Report on the Working of the RBI, 2019-20*. August 2020. Part I.1. pp. 7–9. Accessed at: https://m.rbi.org.in/Scripts/Annual ReportPublications.aspx?year=2020
[29]Ibid., p. 9

capacities, the complete shutdown, as in India, has meant that these capacities were unavailable. The disruption caused to the economy by COVID-19 shutdown mimics that caused by all-out war during World War II.

Modern macroeconomics responded to that experience of wartime uncertainty by developing new theories that justified public investment and public spending. Nation states also responded by creating institutions, such as the Marshall Plan, the International Bank for Reconstruction and Development, and a new multilateral trading system that restored cross-border trade disrupted by war. The major difference between the economic impact of World War II and that of the COVID-19 pandemic is that despite the disruption of normal social and economic activity caused by the war, wartime demand kept economic engines moving. Rather than cater to civilian demand, many industries catered to war demand. With the pandemic lockdown, however, there has been no such trade-off, with overall aggregate demand shrinking.

A second difference between the experience during World War II and now could be that at the end of the war, the restoration of peace and public investment in post-war reconstruction generated optimism about the future and contributed to a speedy recovery of aggregate demand. Within a decade after the war, European economies, including Germany and Italy, as well as the US saw a sharp increase in economic activity. While the end of war in itself generated optimism about the future, the creation of an institutional framework at the national and international level to revive investment, generate employment and stimulate consumption enabled war-torn economies to rapidly re-industrialize and grow.

The economic disruption caused by COVID-19 and the lockdown may not have been as devastating as the economic destruction caused by the great wars, but there are valid parallels.

The sharp drop in maritime trade, the loss of gainful employment and the shortage of goods and services had a debilitating impact on lives and livelihoods. The lockdown too has had a very disruptive and destructive impact on lives and livelihoods, confidence in the future and hence reduced investment and consumption, a loss of gainful employment, and a disruption of internal and maritime trade due to movement restrictions and so forth.

The question today is what would it take for optimism to return to the market so that consumption rises and so do employment and investment. Ending uncertainty about the future and generating positive expectations will remain the biggest policy challenge for most governments. In India, that challenge would be doubly so given the fact that the economy had been slowing down even before the pandemic, with the accumulation of NPAs, a decline in investment rate, rising tariffs, reduced exports and an overall environment of uncertainty. Investors were beginning to believe that between slowing domestic and global demand, the Indian economy would not be able to return very easily and early to the 8 per cent growth trajectory of the 2003–12 period.

◆

I conducted a simple test to judge how expectations about India's potential growth have been altered by the uncertainty gripping investors, employees and consumers. Consider the fact that the economy has been on a rising trajectory of growth over the past half century. The average annual rate of growth for the period 1950–1980 was 3.5 per cent, for 1980–2000 it was 5.5 per cent and for the period 2000–2015 it was around 7.5 per cent, with the economy recording over 8 per cent rate of growth every year between 2004 and 2009. Positive expectations about India's potential growth were shaped by these trends. While there has been a deceleration in the rate of growth of investment and national income in recent years, expectations about future growth potential have remained robust.

In the run-up to the general elections of 2019, the opposition political parties tried to focus public attention on the weakening economic and employment situation. Worried that this might hurt its re-election prospects, the ruling BJP kept its campaign firmly focused on whipping up nationalist sentiment. Yet, one could suggest that until around 2015, the consensus view was that India was on an upward growth trajectory and India's potential growth was seen to be over 7 per cent. When PM Narendra Modi claimed that by 2024 India would be a $5 trillion economy, most viewed it as a credible goal, given that in 2019 the economy was marginally below $3 trillion.

To check how the COVID pandemic and the lockdown may have impacted public perception about growth prospects, I conducted two simple Twitter surveys, the first on 11 August 2020 and the second on 9 September 2020. The question asked was: What average annual rate of growth ought to be forecast for the period 2020–30, given the lockdown and the economic slowdown. In the first round, we offered a choice among four alternative numbers: 5.5 per cent, 6 per cent, 6.5 per cent and 7 per cent. A total of 269 of my over 5,000 Twitter followers responded and voted. As many as 35 per cent of the respondents ticked 5.5 per cent, while 34 per cent ticked 7 per cent. This binary divide can be explained as a political choice, since my Twitter followers are not economists but would have their political biases. Of the remaining 31 per cent, 19 per cent opted for a growth rate of 6 per cent and the remaining 12 per cent ticked 6.5 per cent. All these forecasts are below the peak period growth rate of over 8 per cent during 2004–09, suggesting that expectations regarding India's future growth rate had been considerably moderated.

The second round was conducted on 9 September, after unimpressive data on the 2020–21 first quarter (April–June) GDP was released. The question was the same: the choice offered was between growth rates of 4 per cent, 5 per cent, 6 per cent and 7 per cent. By 9 September, my Twitter followers had increased to 5,982 and of these, 928 responded. Twenty-nine per cent voted for 4 per cent growth, 16 per cent each for 5 per cent and 6 per cent, and 39 per cent opted to vote for 7 per cent. Those familiar with Indian Twitter are aware that both the BJP and the Congress have an army of trolls who would respond to such tweets. Hence, one must discount for such biases in response. However, both polls show that a significant number of respondents see future growth below the trend rate of the pre-COVID period, which would be closer to 7 per cent.

I also sought out the views of a few eminent economists with policy experience in government, including a few who are presently advising the Modi government. The number offered by this informed group was within a wider range of 3.5 per cent to 6.5 per cent. However, a majority forecasted a rate of 6 per cent. Taking the popular public view from Twitter and the informed expert view from my survey, one can hazard the view that expectations of potential growth over the next decade hover around 6 per cent. These purely subjective forecasts of potential future growth contrast with estimates of point-to-point compound annual growth rate (CAGR) for previous decades and a forecast for the period 2020–2030 (Table 2). The forecast for 2020–30 is based on the assumption that in 2020–21 the economy would contract by (-)8.5 per cent. Some may regard this assumption as overly negative. If the contraction is only (-)5 per cent or (-)6 per cent, as suggested by some in government, the end-to-end CAGR would be above 5 per cent, but unlikely to be 6 per cent.

TABLE 2
Real GDP Growth Rates, 1951–2030

Year	1951–52 to 1960–61	1961–62 to 1970–71	1971–72 to 1980–81	1981–82 to 1990–91	1991–92 to 2000–01	2001–02 to 2010–11	2011–12 to 2019–20	2020–21 to 2029–30
CAGR	4.1%	3.9%	3.1%	5.4%	5.9%	6.7%	6.4%	4.24

Source: Personal Correspondence with Omkar Goswami

A growth rate of 6 per cent or less over the next decade would mean that it will take longer for India to be a $5 trillion economy than earlier hoped for. Faced with the sharp downturn in key economic indicators, senior government spokespersons have already shifted goalposts. While the union minister for commerce and industry, Piyush Goyal, claimed as recently as in July 2020 that India would be a $5 trillion economy by 2025 and $10 trillion by 2030, no other senior economic policymaker in government has made such a claim since after the presentation of the union budget in February 2020.[30] A loss of confidence in the growth potential of the economy would mean various economic agents would rework their plans for the future, thereby ensuring that reduced expectations have a way of being fulfilled by reduced performance, which in turn may reduce future expectations. This vicious cycle can only be broken by state intervention and a new policy discourse that emphasizes the centrality of economic growth and development over and above all other political objectives of the political party in government.

◆

---

[30] Piyush Goyal. (2020, July 8). 'Will make India a 10 trillion economy by 2030'. ET Now TV, Accessed at: https://economictimes.indiatimes.com/news/economy/policy/will-make-india-a-10-trillion-economy-by-2030-piyush-goyal/videoshow/76852497.cms?from=mdr

It would be simplistic to assume that uncertainty about economic growth, prospects for future income and employment, and decisions pertaining to consumption, savings and investment are influenced only by economic parameters and economic policy instruments. Expectations about the future are shaped by a wide variety of factors. Economists tend to focus on economic variables but markets, as Keynes reminded us, are moved equally by animal spirits, not reason alone.

Summing up his survey of the Keynesian interpretation of 'animal spirits', Roger Koppl concludes: 'Keynes argued that since entrepreneurs and investors would often be immobilized if they sought to make rational economic decisions, animal spirits are needed to leapfrog rationality and bolster the economy.'[31] COVID has certainly 'immobilized' 'rational' decision-makers and uncertainty has blunted rationality and reason. Investors, savers, consumers, bankers and all economic agents become open to a range of influences—cultural, social, political and economic—that then have consequences for economic decision-making. A pandemic, like war, makes economic agents not just risk-averse but takes them into the realm of uncertainty about future income flows, employment prospects, health costs and so on.

Hence, an important objective of macroeconomic policy has to be to unleash animal spirits bottled up by uncertainty. To revive their animal spirits so that sentiment and expectations turn positive, a government must go beyond supply-side policies and address the problem of uncertain income flows, unemployment, and the threat of unemployment and the consequent risk-aversion that this promotes. These in turn contribute to a reduction in consumption and investment. While pumping hard cash through fiscal and monetary measures can inject liquidity, the challenge

---

[31]Roger Koppl. (1991). 'Animal Spirits', *Journal of Economic Perspectives*, Volume 5, Number 3. p. 209. Accessed at: https://pubs.aeaweb.org/doi/pdf/10.1257/jep.5.3.203

for policy is to weaken the sway of the precautionary motive and encourage households and firms to consume and invest. In that sense, the post-pandemic economy has all the characteristics of a depression economy in which it is demand that would beget supply rather than the other way round.

Many have urged the government to spend more to be able to stimulate both consumption and investment demand, but state intervention has to go beyond fiscal measures. The key to the rising rates of investment that drove higher growth rates in the period 1991–2015 was a combination of positive expectations and animal spirits. Growth in this period was driven by private investment. Going forward, the revival and acceleration of growth will require increased public investment and spending. The government has to recreate the institutions that can facilitate long-term finance and planned public investment, such as development financial institutions and the Planning Commission, respectively.

Economic growth does not occur in a political, social and national security vacuum. Hence, the extant economic slowdown and uncertainty created by COVID cannot be countered through economic instruments alone. Even if policymakers get the fiscal deficit, interest rate, exchange rate, tax and tariff policy right, growth may still remain subdued if uncertainty about the future is plagued by social unrest and the threat of internal and external conflict. It is not a coincidence that periods of higher-than-average growth have been associated with relative political stability at home and peace in our neighbourhood. On the other hand, the past few years of slowing growth have been marked by rising domestic, social and political strife and, more recently, increased geopolitical and security concerns. China's actions along the border may well have been aimed at raising India's political risk and prolonging the uncertainty created by the lockdown.

Hence, the political management of uncertainty is as important as its economic management. How the government deals with domestic, cross-border and regional security challenges is as important to the management of economic uncertainty as reassuring consumers, savers and investors through the tweaking of various policy instruments. It should not be forgotten that the trigger for the 1991 BoP crisis was in fact a spike in India's political risk, rather than concerns about fiscal and payments risks.[32] The latter gained prominence as analysts began to link poor economic management to political factors. The political risk of 1991 was the weakness of unstable coalition governments. The political risk of recent years has been the exact opposite—the uncertainty generated by the actions of a stable government.

◆

Sanjaya Baru is distinguished fellow at the Manohar Parrikar Institute for Defence Studies and Analyses and the United Service Institution of India. He has been the chief editor of *The Financial Express* and *Business Standard*, and media advisor to the PM of India. He was also the director for Geo-economic and Strategy at the International Institute of Strategic Studies, UK (2011–16).

---

[32]For more on this proposition, see Sanjaya Baru. (2016). *1991: How P.V. Narasimha Rao Made History*, Aleph Book Company, New Delhi. pp. 40–43

THE FISCAL DIMENSION

TOWARDS A NEW FRAMEWORK FOR FEDERALISM

Haseeb A. Drabu

The COVID-19 pandemic has exposed the fault lines of federalism in India like never before. The policy responses to the unprecedented crisis have not only lacked in coordination, and even worked at cross purposes, but have also failed to leverage the strengths of the three levels of governance. Indeed, it reached a point where the management of the pandemic has become a Centre-versus-states issue. There is little doubt that the pandemic has exposed the union government's commitment to a federal constitutional republic to a degree unmatched since its birth. This has become possible because the foundational framework of federalism and its design as laid out in the Constitution of India is not just weak but outdated.

In dealing with the pandemic, what has contributed to the conflict between the Centre and the states is that the union government has relied on presumed authority rather than on its constitutional mandate and the evolved practice. This has resulted in the under-leveraging of the deep and diversified democratic institutional infrastructures and their network, which has been created over the last 70 years. Seen in this context, federalism, which should have been a strength, has been made out to be a weakness, laying the ground for a further greater centralization of the decision-making system in the country. As such, the pandemic occasions a serious national debate about what a competent and well-functioning federal democracy should stand for and how it should manage its routine affairs and situation of crisis.

In this essay, it is suggested that the current federal framework, which is colonial in its moorings, unionist in its ideology and patriarchal in its operations, needs a complete rethink. Its instrumentalities, which have evolved in the context of a closed command economy, have to be redesigned to suit the needs of an open regulated economy. The scope and remit of federalism have to be widened to include the newer forms of government intervention aligned to the new economic structure. In the new framework, the Centre should exercise leadership instead of control, and economic support instead of dominance. It is this that should form the basis of the new federal compact of the union with the states.

This is all the more important in the context of a distinct move from a republican democracy to a majoritarian one, which has far-reaching implications and consequences for the Indian nation and the nation state—be it the social compact with the people across the country or the political–economic compact with states in the union.

Even though the nature of economic regime has changed completely since 1991, the institutional landscape of federalism has been altered and the fiscal relations between the Centre and state governments have undergone major changes, especially in the recent years. The framework of federalism in the country has remained unchanged. In order to make it relevant and effective, the framework of fiscal federalism needs to be redesigned for an open regulated economy.

The needs, requirements and policy instrumentalities of an open regulated economy are very different from those of a closed economy for which the framework has been designed. The central government was the principal driver for growth and development through public investment, which was financed by raising the level of domestic savings. Seven decades later, the situation is radically different. The public investment-led growth, strategy has been replaced by a private investment-driven growth helped by a liberalized domestic and foreign investment regime. In the mid-1980s, out of the total gross domestic capital formation in the economy, 60 per cent was contributed by the public sector. This is down to around 20 per cent now. Almost 80 per cent of gross domestic fixed capital formation is now generated by the private sector. The non-governmental financial flows have dwarfed the gross transfer of revenues from the Centre to the states: at ₹12 trillion it is less than 15 per cent of the financial flows from the banking segment alone. If the allocations of institutional finance and capital market flows are added to this, the share of government flows would be in single digits. Yet, as a hangover of the controlled closed economy, the literature on fiscal federalism continues to focus on transfers from the Centre to the states.

Regulatory Federalism

The demise of the old control and command state has seen the rise of the new regulatory state in India—equally centralized, more pervasive and all-powerful. Post-1991, there has been a proliferation of 'autonomous' regulatory institutions set up under acts of Parliament in various sectors and spheres of the national and state economies. To a large extent, the direct ministerial and bureaucratic control has been replaced by indirect regulatory diktat. This regulatory state, as it is today, is nothing but an extended arm of the central government; not only in terms of control, but even in their design, the regulatory bodies are extremely union-centric. In most cases, apart from the template of regulation that has been designed, drafted and distributed by the Centre, even the people who are manning these bodies are from the central government. More often than not, the Centre's reluctance to cede the control that it had in the earlier regime has meant that the regulators are fighting battles not with the regulated entities but with the central government for clarity and control. This has major ramifications for the possibility of effective regulation.

The states have very little role in this crucial area of public policy. The authority to set the regulatory standards rests with the Centre, while the state governments have to just report or, at best, monitor compliance. They don't even have the authority to choose the combination of policies to meet the set standards. It is a well-established research finding that this form of delegation tends to be the least efficient form. In fact, the reverse form of delegation, in which state governments choose their own individual standards, which the central government then decides how to collectively adhere to, is seen to be the most efficient.

The network of these regulatory authorities cuts into the ambit of the federal powers of policymaking at various levels. Indeed, the Centre has found it as the least controversial route to make inroads into the state list. This not only raises serious concerns regarding the vertical division of regulatory power, but also the misalignment between the state and central governments. The differing objectives and incentives undermine the very purpose of the regulatory statutes.

With regard to the manner in which the country is shaping up, it is important to federalize the regulatory setup only if to break the new congruence of powers—executive, legislative and judicial—within the regulatory system. It is instructive to study the IBC process in the country wherein the Supreme Court is now functioning like a resolution professional in the stressed asset space.

In a political regime with overwhelming electoral majority, the regulators chosen are turning out to be the pliant and political bureaucrats and judges, leading to a complete capture of the regulatory setup. In fact, that is one of the biggest dangers facing the country today. Increasingly, there are no autonomous bodies.

There is need to develop a model of regulatory federalism that lays out the authority to set the standard, and the authority to choose the combination of policies to meet the standard should be allocated between the central government and the state governments. In any efficient system of regulation, there has to be a delegation of regulated authority: the central government may retain the power to either set or meet the standard, but not both, and delegate the power to make the remaining decision to the state governments. The issue of how to distribute regulatory power between the two tiers of government must be formulated comprehensively.

Resource Federalism

This leads to the second key issue for new federalism in India—natural resources, which is the focus area of the regulatory state. In a market-led growth paradigm, natural resources—minerals, oil, gas and water—are the key revenue drivers for, and major constraints to, macroeconomic growth and its spread across the subnational economies. In the extant system, this resource dimension is absent from the scheme of federal transfers. Indeed, even a rational framework for the redistribution of resource rents (the compensation to states on this account is many times that of the GST compensation that states are currently agitating for!) is yet to evolve. Not only are the financial transfers independent of the contribution by a region to the commodity-deficient national economy, but the central government also corners a disproportionately large part of the revenues emanating from these. In the case of minerals, for instance, iron ore, states receive a meagre 20 per cent share in the form of royalty and state GST, while the Centre's share, mainly from income and dividend tax, is 80 per cent. This is because large profits are made by iron ore companies due to increased demand, high prices and the very low royalty payments that they make to states.

The central government extracts a substantial share of revenue indirectly from these resources. At the pre-production stage, the Centre collects revenue as forest conservation charges and labour welfare cess; in the production stage in the form of custom duty, excise duty, income tax and corporate taxes; and in the post-production stage as central tax and export duty. In addition to this, the central government, through its public sector undertakings, which are the biggest consumers of minerals, has an additional, indirect source of revenues. The Centre has been milking these minerals cows through dividend, and can also monetize their value by divesting its stake in these enterprises. The net result is that distribution of revenues emanating from natural resources is effectively two-thirds in favour of the Centre.

The real challenge going forward is to design a framework for 'resources revenue sharing' in addition to the 'transactional revenue sharing' that has traditionally been done so far. In other words, fiscal federalism must be now linked to resource federalism in India. A new alternative framework can start with a fair scheme for distribution of resource rents, but it must eventually graduate towards a more robust and institutionalized system of resource federalism. In doing so, it would have aligned the existing fiscal federal setup to work in an open regulated market economy. One of the criteria for the quantum of statutory of transfers should be the contribution of a region to the development of natural resources. This is especially important going forward, as India is a resource-deficit economy and there is a premium on raw materials.

To start with, the existing royalty system, which at present is an ad hoc mix of unit-based and ad valorem-based approaches, must be revised and restructured. A move towards a non-discretionary and automatic system of indexed ad valorem rates that moves in line with the commodity price movement needs to be made. It is quite anomalous, for instance, that coal rates, which accounts for the largest share of royalty revenue, have been revised only four or maybe five times since the nationalization of the industry in the early 1970s.

For a long time, resource-rich states have been raising a banner of revolt against the very low royalty given to them under the current revenue repatriation arrangement. In fact, a number of states have reached out to the higher judiciary many times, seeking to raise their share in the revenue pool concerning natural resources. Although several court judgements have come to the rescue of states, this remains a non-starter.

With the states having been deprived of their fair share from resources, there is a palpable resurgence of regionalism that is fuelling protectionism. Whether it is to protect regional businesses or cover up for their loss of governmental revenues, the fact is that there is now a discernible rise in 'subnational protectionism'. For instance, Odisha stipulated that 60 per cent iron ore mined must be used within the state. Karnataka took it upon itself to decide on the actual quantity each iron ore mine can produce and supervise its utilization. Assam legislated levying a cess on the crude removed from its 'domiciled' facilities. Many states are seeking an imposition of Mineral Resource Rent Tax at the rate of 50 per cent of the supernormal profits being made by mine owners. This is a long list and all the new levies, be it in the form of an entry tax, an extraction cess or export duty, are in addition to existing taxes/duties by the state and not in line with the overall direction of tax regime that the country is moving towards. Left unaddressed, the administrative boundaries of a state will slowly but surely be converted into an economic border. This flies in the face of a single unified common market of common economic space, which is being created by the new indirect tax regime—the GST.

Post-GST Fiscal Federalism

As such, it has become imperative to relook at the entire framework of federalism post the introduction of GST as a tax regime. The fundamental change in tax regime must appropriately inform the redesign of fiscal federalism. The manner in which the union and states have pooled their tax sovereignty ought to be the cornerstone of new federalism in India.

In the post-GST era, the entire concept and criteria of horizontal distribution has to be reviewed. The existing criteria for devolution have been formulated in the context of an origin-based production system of taxation. Now, with GST, it is a destination-based consumption tax regime. Operationally, the earlier taxation system was favourable to the 'producer states'. The new tax regime will benefit the 'consumer states'. How the service tax is contributing to the states' revenue balances is yet to be totally deciphered. Both these will make a significant difference to the need for inter se distribution of equalizing grants. A number of things, including the pecking order of states, are bound to see major reordering and recalibration.

The fact that a large part of the revenue kitty, which the Finance Commission devolves, is now being determined by the GST Council, will have to be factored in, as the distributable pool is no longer the consequence of the central government's unilateral decision. Any decision on the rate bands, for instance, by the GST Council, will have huge implications on the vertical distribution of revenues between the states and the Centre. Even the 'gap-filling' approach through the Article 275 transfers or the 'deficit grants' will have to be redesigned not only in light of the inter se distribution—Integrated GST—but also the compensation law approved by the Parliament. The erstwhile non-plan revenue deficit will now have to be estimated by states as a pre-devolution revenue deficit based on their own tax growth. With a share in central taxes, this gap for states will be covered in part or whole. If a post-devolution revenue deficit persists, the Finance Commission will have to finance it with gap grants but only after the guaranteed compensation.

In light of the pooling of tax sovereignty by the Centre and the states under the GST regime, the new fiscal federal framework should be redesigned as vertical transfers and horizontal distribution exclusively based on revenue sharing. The idea should be to maximize the revenue sharing between the Centre and states, and minimizing the expenditure underwriting of states by the Centre. There should be no expenditure underwriting in the form of scheme and programmes funded by the Centre. The devolution hiked by the 14th Finance Commission should be enough to allow for a reduction in all such expenditure underwriting transfers done by the Centre. This will not only give the states greater flexibility to design programmes but also leave the management of actual gaps to them, making the existing system of vertical transfers neater. This will sow the seeds of a new fiscal federal system.

Apart from fiscal federalism, the creation of a common economic market with GST, a high dispersion value of inflation across regions and its persistence over time can have serious implications on regional wage rates and standard of living, and pose a challenge for subnational policymaking. This brings up the final piece in the model of new federalism—monetary policy.

Monetary Federalism

As of now, monetary policy is completely dominated by the Centre. The RBI, in its architecture, both legislative as well as organizational, is unitary. It has nothing to do with the political constitution of the country. Not surprising then that monetary federalism has rarely, if ever, figured in the discussion on Indian federalism, especially fiscal federalism. In a regulated open economy, the fiscal federal system needs to be complemented by monetary federalism.

The case for looking at monetary federalism at this point is manyfold. For one, in an open economy, monetary policy is the main tool of policy intervention as fiscal interventions have reached their limit. Second, the case for monetary federalism rests on the fact that there is a differential impact of monetary policy on states, depending on the level of their economic development, the financial deepening of the state and the extent of industrialization. Third, unlike in the past, in a market economy, RBI is increasingly being called in to perform developmental roles. Because of a single currency and free factor mobility, prices across states and regions are contemporaneously correlated. Because of the differing structure of subnational economies and their varying levels of development, price levels are affected by local shocks. The RBI is increasingly going to be faced with inter-state and sectoral inflation-related problems.

Finally, of late there have been serious efforts to make the RBI do its bidding in a more structured manner than influencing financial sector policies as was done earlier. For instance, the manner in which the issue of the RBI's reserves and its dividend to the Government of India was handled, resulted in compromising its position and further weakened its already emaciated autonomous decision-making.

Similarly, in 2016, the MPC was set up by amending the RBI Act via the Finance Act (2016). While this was a good development, the procedure adopted for it—the amendment was introduced and passed as a non-money bill to escape the stumbling block of the Opposition-controlled Rajya Sabha—was not just undemocratic but also anti-federal in its moorings as it bypassed the House of States. As it is, the MPC consists of six members—the RBI governor, deputy governor, executive director, plus three independent directors—all nominated by the Government of India. The MPC decides by majority, which really means that it is the Centre deciding it. This can be a political adventure in a very sensitive, technical monetary matter of national and international concerns and with consequences. It has opened the door to politicization and populist interventions.

More importantly, from the perspective of macroeconomic and monetary management, it needs to be recognized that in the new economic regime, the state governments' market borrowings, the main source of funding for their gross fiscal deficits, has increased from less than 10 per cent before 1990 to around 75 per cent now. As a result of this increase, the gross market borrowings of state governments are now budgeted to be similar to that of the central government. The states collectively now borrow around 3 per cent of GDP, which amounts to around ₹5,500 billion. The share of state loans in total outstanding loans has nearly doubled from 15 per cent to 2007–08 to about 30 per cent in 2018–19, while that of the Government of India has declined from 85 per cent to 70 per cent. These structural changes have an obvious bearing on the relationship between subnational governments and the central bank, which goes beyond bilateral agreements and advisory.

This large stock and supply of state development loans (SDLs) has an impact on the yields of central government securities as well as the spreads on corporate bonds. Unlike the central government debt, which crowds out bank credit, SDLs crowd out corporate borrowings in the bond market by increasing costs. It has been observed that a 1 percentage point increase in the ratio of state debt issuance to GDP results in an 11 per cent decline in the volume value of corporate bonds.

Also, by international capital standards, Basel III assigns credit risk weights to sub-sovereign borrowings and when implemented, state governments will need to strategize for this eventuality and so will RBI as the regulator. This cannot be done in the absence of a new subnational financial architecture.

A new system must be put in place where state governments can plan reissuances, buyback and switches based on their respective maturity profiles and cash flows. This will help create volumes, facilitate trading in the secondary market and benefit them by lowering yields. The economic and social welfare of citizens is through a market economy and is dependent on effective fiscal and debt management by the states. Building robust SDL markets and augmenting debt management systems in states to take care of emergent risks is both imperative and urgent.

In the absence of a functional relationship between the states and the central bank, there are hardly any differences in inter-state spreads, with no observed relationship between the spread and the indebtedness of states. As such, states are neither rewarded nor penalized for their fiscal performance, which obviously results in better financially managed states cross-subsidizing the other states. This is akin to financial repression.

While the management of the central government's debt is conducted by the RBI under statutory provisions that oblige the central government to delegate its debt management to the RBI, the debt of the subnational governments, on the other hand, is managed by the RBI under bilateral agreements. The RBI, through a statutory relationship, will be able to hold the state government's borrowing costs to a minimum over the medium to long term, while keeping the associated risks to a prudent level. In the process, a market-oriented subnational debt regime will be created.

On the basis of these factors, there is a prima facie case for repositioning the RBI as a federal central bank. While this needs to be thought through and there have to be safeguards, giving the existing central reserve bank a federal reserve bank character should not be that difficult or disruptive. The first step towards this end would be to reorganize the existing regional boards of the RBI and empower them. At present, they are at best ornamental and, at worst, dysfunctional bodies.

The regional board can be provided with research services, which can enable them to prepare an agenda for discussion at the meetings based on the research of monetary and credit conditions and enterprises in their respective jurisdictions. The discussion at the meeting can thus be well informed and candid and help the governor to take their concerns in the preparation of his six-monthly statement to be presented before Parliament as suggested earlier in this article. Thus, regional and national interests could be made mutually reinforcing.

To start with, the local boards of RBI in Mumbai, Kolkata, Chennai and New Delhi could be federalized. The members of the local boards of RBI are appointed by the central government for a term of four years. This can be changed to involve the state government in the four zones.

Once this is done, the Central Board of RBI, which is empowered to delegate functions to the regional boards, can mandate these regional boards to make policy recommendations on local matters and to represent the territorial and economic interests of local cooperative and indigenous banks. In view of the emerging banking crisis, especially in the cooperative banking sector, the local RBI boards can be asked to play a regulatory role. Why can't the regional boards be mandated to represent regional developmental interests as well?

To conclude, the extant federal framework that functions more as a decentralized model of governance than a fiscal federal model has to be rid of its colonial moorings and closed economy rigidities. It has to be reformulated in the context of an open regulated economy through the widening of its ambit by dividing the regulatory powers between the two tiers of government, sharing not just the tax revenues but the revenues accruing form usage of natural resources, and including states in the formulation of the monetary policy.

In this new scheme of federalism, it might be a good idea to move away from the overwhelming dominance of the structure of 'vertical federalism' inbuilt in the Indian model of federalism—a one-way traffic from the Centre to the states. The way in which it has been structured precludes individual states from coordinating and sharing powers with each other. It might well be time to introduce 'lateral federalism' in the fiscal-federal policy regime in India. If individual states coordinate with each other, then they could internalize externalities and achieve the social optimum for the federation.

◆

Haseeb Drabu is former minister of finance, Government of Jammu and Kashmir, and former chairman, Jammu & Kashmir Bank. He has worked at the Indian Planning Commission and Finance Commission.

PREPARE FOR STRESS AND PAIN

Omkar Goswami

On 31 August 2020, the Government of India released its GDP and GVA estimates for April–June 2020 (Q1 FY21). Battered by COVID-19, the numbers were predictably dismal. Real GDP growth had contracted by 23.9 per cent versus the same quarter last year, and real GVA growth was almost as bad at (-)22.8 per cent. With very limited buffers, the pandemic has hurt the informal sector more than others, and until there are more detailed estimates of the informal sector, these numbers remain provisional. The scenario could be worse.

This crunch was expected by all. Unfortunately, India was going through a period of steadily deteriorating GDP growth well before COVID-19 and the nationwide lockdown that was imposed from 25 March till 31 May 2020. The last bright quarter was January–March 2018 (Q4 FY19), when India clocked real GDP growth of 8.2 per cent. As Chart 1 shows, it has been downhill since then, with growth dwindling to lacklustre rates.

Thus, before exploring what our post-COVID growth rates might be over the next few years and advocating reforms for a more vibrant economy, we need to understand why growth slowed the way it did pre-COVID, and whether the factors inhibiting growth in the pre-disease era will remain, intensify or serendipitously fade away in the near term.

A close look at the GDP data suggests some seriously disturbing trends. It is useful to start with GFCF, which shows

Chart 1: Real GDP Growth

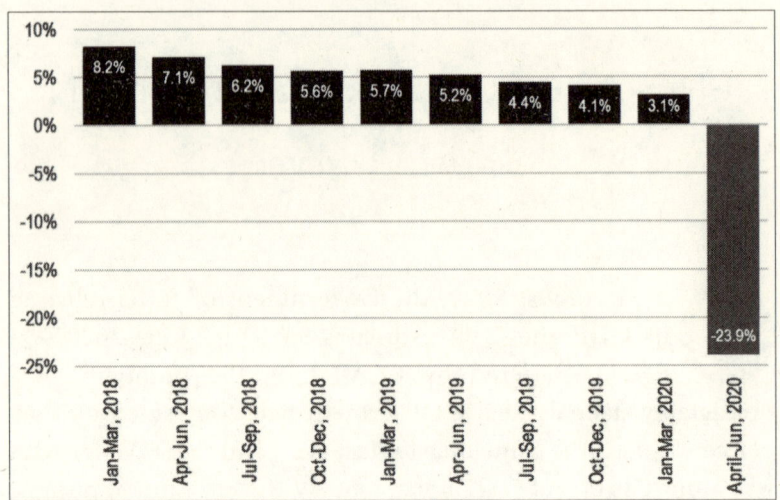

Source: Unless stated otherwise, all GDP-based data is from the Ministry of Statistics and Programme Implementation, Government of India.

how much of new value added in an economy is invested for future output, rather than consumed.

In July–September 2011, GFCF as a share of GDP was 35.6 per cent. That was creditable: during the year, compared to other Asian nations, only China had a higher ratio. Since then, however, it has been heading south, a decline that began with the deterioration in construction and real estate. For three successive quarters leading up to 31 March 2020, GFCF fell to below 30 per cent of GDP. The denouement has come in April–June 2020, with the ratio dropping to 22.3 per cent, which is by far the lowest that India has seen since 1997–98. Chart 2.A plots the declining share of GFCF to GDP; and Chart 2.B plots the precipitous fall in the rates of growth of both GDP and GFCF. Together, these say a simple story: we were weakening well before Q1 FY21, after which COVID-19 and the lockdown delivered a body blow.

Chart 2A: Falling share of GFCF in GDP

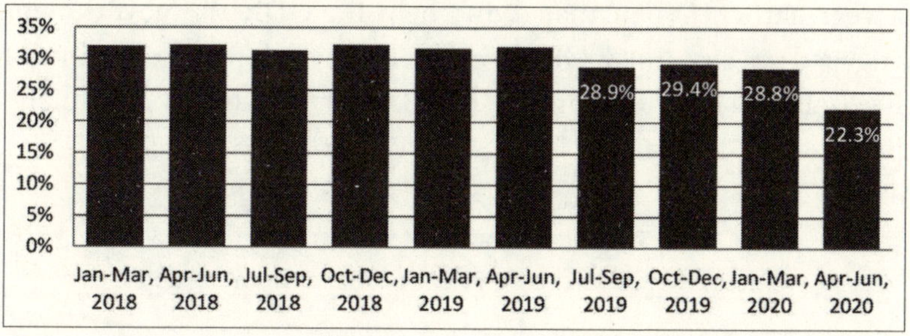

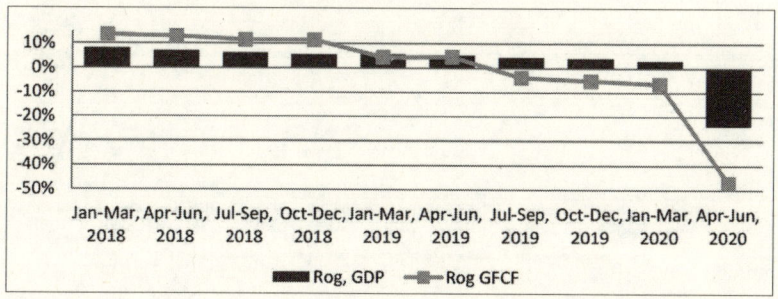

Chart 2B: Falling growth of GDP and GFCF

By 2019–20, therefore, GFCF, a key spark plug of growth, wasn't firing. Neither was another spark plug: private final consumer expenditure (PFCE). Between 2000–01 and 2016–17, PFCE rose impressively, thanks to the growth of retail and consumer loans from banks and NBFCs, and created a boom for cars, two-wheelers, refrigerators, colour TV sets and other consumer durables. Then it started to slow down. From a high of 8.8 per cent in Q2 FY19, growth of PFCE started steadily decreasing until it hit 2.7 per cent in Q4 FY20. In April–June 2020, this growth collapsed to (-)26.7 per cent.

In recent times, the union government has tried to counteract the flagging GFCF and PFCE growth by substantially increasing the government's final consumption expenditure (GFCE) via the exchequer. In Q4 FY19, real GFCE grew by 14.4 per cent versus a year earlier. When that didn't help lift GDP, the government engaged in sustained GFCE increases: by 14.2 per cent in Q2 FY20, by 13.4 per cent in Q3, by 13.6 per cent in Q4 and finally by 16.4 per cent in Q1 FY21. Chart 3 plots the data.

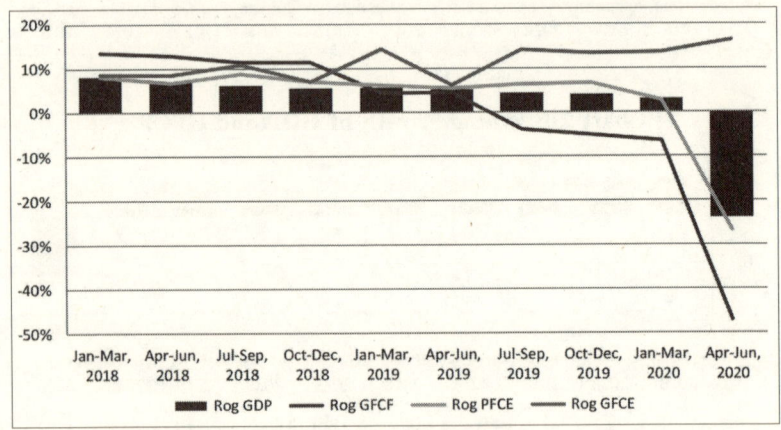

Chart 3: Determinants of declining growth

The chart is instructive, for it shows:

1. How real GFCF growth has been falling over the last 10 successive quarters.
2. How real PFCE growth has been dropping over the last seven quarters.
3. How the government tried to compensate by raising GFCE, especially over the last four quarters.
4. How the government's dramatic increases of GFCE in recent times have not borne fruit. GDP growth continued to fall to reach 3.1 per cent in January–March 2020, the slowest growth since quarterly data was available from 2004, after which came the COVID-19 cataclysm.

India in the COVID World

As I write this in mid-September 2020, the world has witnessed over 28 million certified COVID-19 cases, with the US, India and Brazil leading the pack. Though we have a low fatality rate of 1.7 per cent, versus over 3 per cent for both the US and Brazil and 10.8 per cent for Mexico, there are some seriously worrying trends in India.

Despite a large base, some 4 million certified COVID-positive cases across the country, the cumulative number is increasing at an extremely high exponential trend rate of 3.3 per cent per day—one that is significantly higher than that in the US (1.3 per cent) or Brazil (2.2 per cent). These days, the typical daily rise in confirmed cases veers between 80,000 and 90,000. This is why we have already overtaken Brazil to become the second-worst COVID-affected country in the world. At these rates of growth, we could even surpass the US soon. Chart 4 plots the data.

Furthermore, the disease is spreading rapidly to different parts of India. Earlier, it was concentrated in Maharashtra, Delhi and partly Gujarat. Thereafter, it has proliferated across several other states: Tamil Nadu is now the second worst after Maharashtra, followed by Andhra Pradesh, Tamil Nadu, Karnataka, Uttar Pradesh, Delhi, West Bengal, Bihar and Telangana.

Consequently, each state's and district's administration is doing what it thinks is best to contain the disease. Most of these are haphazard with one economically damaging commonality: arbitrary lockdowns of different durations when confronted by high caseloads.

I stress lockdowns for two reasons. First, COVID will remain with us through the first quarter of 2021, if not longer, and will conflagrate across different geographies over the coming period. Second, until an affordable vaccine is introduced and made universally available in India, which is unlikely till the end of

Chart 4: The spread of COVID-19

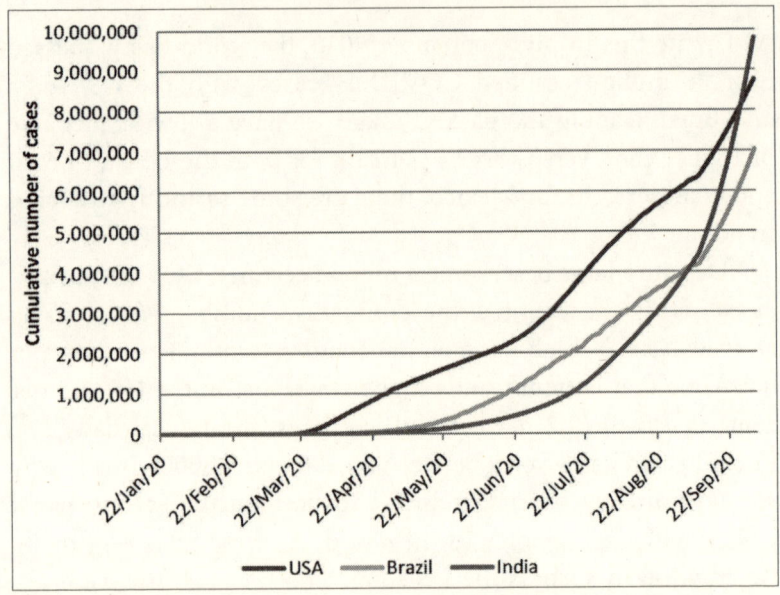

Source: For the US and Brazil, from Johns Hopkins Coronavirus Research Center (coronavirus.jhu.edu). For India, from covid19india.org.

the first half of 2021, the inevitable response to infection spikes will be local, district-wise or state-wise lockdowns.[33] These will continue wreaking damage to the economy until well after the first half of 2020–21.

---

[33] As of end August 2020, all districts of Punjab had weekend lockdowns from 6 pm on Saturday to 9 am on Monday. All districts of Uttar Pradesh were locked down every weekend. All districts in Bihar were under full lockdown until 6 September 2020. In Maharashtra, 19 municipal corporations were under varying forms of lockdown. Tamil Nadu had imposed complete lockdowns on Sundays. West Bengal had done so for two arbitrary days per week. In all, 345 of India's 734 districts, involving over 53 per cent of the population, were in some form of lockdown or another.
Hindustan Times. (26 August 2020). 'Curbs for 53% of India'. New Delhi edition, p.4

GDP Growth: Estimate for 2020–21 (FY21) and up to 2023–24 (FY24)

Let me now put forward an estimate of real GDP growth for 2020–21, which requires making assumptions about quarterly growth during the year.

a) Q1 2020–21 was a washout, with real GDP growth crashing to (-)23.9 per cent. I have assumed that after the revisions incorporate more informal sector data than the provisional estimate, GDP growth for the quarter will be (-)25 per cent.

b) A sputtering start worsened by a series of state-level lockdowns should also affect GDP growth for Q2. My estimate is (-)15 per cent.

c) Thereafter, we should see some signs of pickup. However, despite that, Q3 FY21 will still see GDP growth shrinking by 7.5 per cent compared to the same quarter of the previous year.

d) Finally, I have assumed GDP growth for Q4 FY21 at (-)5 per cent.

Based on these estimates, my forecast for annual GDP growth in 2020–21 is (-)12.9 per cent. It could be worse, depending upon how muted the performance is in the second half of the year.

Thanks to the lower base at the end of FY21, I have assumed a bounceback of 8 per cent growth for FY22, followed by 5.5 per cent growth for both FY23 and FY24. What this translates to is given in Table 1.

TABLE 1
Forecast of real GDP growth, FY20 to FY24

	GDP growth (annual)	GDP (normalized)
2019–20	4.2%	1000
2020–21 (F)	-12.9%	87.10
2021–22 (F)	8%	947
2022–23 (F)	5.5%	99.24
2023–24 (F)	5.5%	104.70
CAGR		
Using end-points	1.1%	
Semi-log trend rate	2.2%	

Source: Government of India, CSO, Ministry of Statistics and Programme Implementation, national income data, quarterly and annual.

Note: (F) is forecast.

These growth rates suggest a dire situation. Even after a natural rebound in 2021–22, India's real GDP will be lower than what it was in 2019–20. And the CAGR over the next four years should be between 1.1 per cent (using end-points) and 2.2 per cent (semi-log trend rate)—rates that are wholly insufficient for the need of the nation.

Why do these numbers look so bleak? To understand that, we must again look at the various determinants of growth.

Again, GFCF is a good place to start. COVID and the lockdown have led to virtually all enterprises drastically cutting expenditure and holding on to hard-earned cash. The corporate sector had seriously slowed down on investments over the last three years. It will be foolhardy to expect any meaningful investment rebound either in FY21 or FY22. Facing a lack of demand and severe excess capacities, corporates will maximize their cash, cut costs everywhere and try to generate productivity improvements without investing in additional plant and machinery. This is a given over the next two years.

Hence, the share of GFCF to GDP will decline over the four quarters of FY21. It fell to 22.3 per cent in Q1, which was a huge decline of 9.7 percentage points. I expect this to be the same in Q2. Thereafter, it might marginally rise to 24 per cent and 25 per cent in Q3 and Q4, respectively.

If so, then in annual terms, the share of GFCF to GDP will have deteriorated by 6.2 percentage points between FY20 and FY21, from 29.8 per cent to 23.5 per cent. Thus, the ratio of GFCF to GDP will decline yet again after hitting a 13-year low in FY20.

Unfortunately, post-COVID expenditure patterns suggest that households, too, are conserving cash. That is expected and wholly understandable. Families are worried about the continuity of livelihood. Barring bare essential durables that couldn't be bought in Q1 2020–21, they are keeping a tight lid on household expenditure and saving wherever they can. This also shows up in the data.

In absolute terms, real PFCE has reduced by 27 per cent in Q1 FY20 and the ratio of PFCE to GDP dropped by 2.1 percentage points to 54.3 per cent—the lowest in 11 successive quarters. Between the period ending 28 February 2020 and 31 July 2020, aggregate deposits of all SCBs increased by 6.3 per cent. In contrast, bank credit rose by just 1.5 per cent over the same period. COVID has not only forced both households and firms to consume less and save more, but has also reduced lending opportunities for banks, which are in any case saddled by a large stock of non-performing loans. In such circumstances, it is wishful to expect any kick-start to PFCE across all four quarters of FY21 and probably going into FY22.

This leaves GFCE. Unfortunately, there are limits to increasing government expenditure with a creaking exchequer.

That is precisely why Finance Minister Nirmala Sitharaman's

economic revival package of mid-May 2020 totting up to ₹20,971 billion (₹21 lakh crore or 10.3 per cent of nominal GDP) had a direct fiscal outgo of only ₹2,135 billion (₹2,13,500 crore), or a tad below 1 per cent of GDP. The financial cost of much of the package—to the extent of it actually being incurred—is being borne by public sector banks and the RBI.

State of the Central Exchequer in FY21

One should expect the fiscal cupboard to be well-nigh empty in FY21. COVID has brought about a massive fall in both the GST and direct tax revenues. This shortfall will persist throughout the year. Given below are my estimates leading up to the revenue, primary and fiscal deficits for 2020–21.

a) Tax revenue (net to the Centre) will be down by 30 per cent—by almost ₹491,000 crore—compared to the budget estimate (BE) of 2020–21. That implies a hit of 2.37 per cent of GDP.[34]

b) Non-tax revenue will reduce by 20 per cent vs. BE 2020–21, or by ₹77,000 crore—translating to 0.37 per cent of GDP.

c) Therefore, revenue receipts will be down by 2.74 per cent of GDP.

d) The ambitious divestment target of ₹210,000 crore in BE 2020–21 will not be met by a long shot. At best, we can hope for ₹105,000 crore, or 50 per cent of the target. Thus, on disinvestment alone, there will be an extra shortfall of 0.51 per cent of GDP.

e) Moreover, there could be a 10 per cent increase in

---

[34] In BE 2020–21, nominal GDP was expected to grow by 10 per cent to ₹22,489,420 crore. Given an estimated fall in real GDP of 12.9 per cent compensated by an annual inflation of 5 per cent, I have assumed nominal GDP to fall by 7.9 per cent. That is the denominator for all the GDP-based ratios.

revenue expenditure over BE 2020–21. That would be an additional 1.27 per cent of GDP.
f) Hence, I expect the Centre's revenue deficit (total revenue expenditure less revenue receipts) to rise from 2.7 per cent of GDP in BE 2020–21 to 7 per cent of GDP.
g) The fiscal deficit will balloon from an estimated 3.5 per cent of GDP in BE 2020–21 to 8.4 per cent.
h) And the primary deficit (fiscal deficit-less interest payments) will burgeon from a BE of 0.4 per cent of GDP to 4.9 per cent.

With an eye to capping the fiscal deficit, the union government will doubtless do all it can to garner non-tax revenues. But there are limits to that in FY21. Given the terrible state of most state-owned enterprises and the weight of non-performing loans of public sector banks, there is only so much that can be achieved by demanding higher dividends. Even before COVID, the divestment target seemed super-ambitious. Today, it is virtually impossible to achieve.

Having said so, I expect the Finance Ministry to go in a collection overdrive: through dividend and special payments from the RBI, though these cannot be as much as in FY20; through so-called divestments, where dominant state-owned financial undertakings such as the Life Insurance Corporation of India, the government-owned general insurance corporations and some major banks will be 'persuaded' to buy shares of central public sector enterprises; and by compelling public sector undertakings to ante up 36 per cent higher dividends—as put out in the receipts budget for FY21—even at the cost of depleting corporate reserves.

The GST Compensation Cess: A Crisis of Fiscal Federalism

Without doubt, the collapse of GST revenue is the most important fiscal problem facing the central government. It began in FY20 and has dramatically worsened since then. This has not only badly affected tax revenues but also created a serious trust deficit in fiscal federalism through the GST Compensation Cess (or Comp Cess). It needs explaining.

The 'carrot' to secure the assent of all states to a nation-wide GST was to assure them that over five years beginning July 2017, if a state's indirect tax revenue from GST increased at less than a CAGR of 14 per cent calculated from a base year of 2015–16, the difference would be made good by the union. It was doubtless a large carrot offered by the then finance minister, Arun Jaitley, to get the states on board. The Comp Cess—levied at different rates on 21 goods such as paan masala, gutkha, tobacco products, aerated water, motor vehicles and the like—was set up for collecting this money.

Things went well for the first two years, when the Comp Cess revenue exceeded what was necessary to recompense the states. When the economy started faltering in FY20, GST revenues fell as did the Comp Cess collection. Suddenly, the 14 per cent promise looked too expensive.[35] Then came COVID and the nationwide lockdown. The piggy bank was busted.

In a GST Council meeting on 27 August 2020, Finance Minister Nirmala Sitharaman stated that the Comp Cess shortfall for 2020–21 would be ₹2.35 crore. After citing the Attorney General's opinion that the Centre had no legal obligation to borrow to pay this shortfall to the states, she offered two unpalatable options.

Under option 1, states could borrow from the RBI up to ₹97,000 crore, which she claimed was the shortfall purely on account of GST implementation. The rest of the gap, according to her, was an 'act of God' for which she asserted that no payment is required by law.

---

[35] Even so, the Centre paid the states at 14 per cent growth for 2019–20. However, each of these payments was delayed.

Under option 2, states could borrow the full shortfall of ₹2.35 lakh crore, for which the Centre was willing to relax the borrowing threshold under the FRBM Act, 2003.

All non-BJP-ruled states have rallied against this as a failure in the terms of agreement, and have insisted that the Centre should borrow to make good the shortfall. I believe this to be logically true; more so given the ethical compass of fiscal federalism. The Centre fashioned a constitutional deal for a five-year period to make good any revenue shortfall to the states. That period continues. So, the deficit should be made good by the Centre's borrowings.

This is best explained in simple English: If I undertake to pay you ₹1,000 every year for five years and I can't meet it, then I ought to borrow to make good that promise. I might even say, 'I can't give you ₹1,000 in one go. May I give it in two instalments?' But I definitely can't say, 'Sorry, *I'm* broke. So, why don't *you* borrow to cover the dues that *I'm* obliged to pay?'

Each state has one vote in the GST Council. With the BJP controlling the majority of states, it is likely that the council will opt for the first option. That doesn't make it any less morally repugnant. It is a deeply worrying imbroglio that is being played out at the high altar of fiscal federalism. In the short run, the central government may come up as a 'winner'. But it will be a pyrrhic victory. After this, no state will trust any fiscal concord with the union. Indeed, I fear that the very future of the GST is at stake.

Irrespective of the Comp Cess problem, there are severe challenges to GST revenues. Even in FY20, total GST revenue including Comp Cess was just 3.8 per cent higher than the previous year.[36] April 2020 was a disaster with GST revenue at

---

[36]If March 2020 revenues were to be ignored on account of the first seven days of the nationwide lockdown, the 11-month collection (April–February) of 2019–20 was only 5 per cent higher than the same 11 months of 2018–19.

28.3 per cent versus April 2019. Things have improved since then: May 2020 GST revenue was at 62 per cent compared to the same month in the previous year, June 2020 was at 91 per cent, July 2020 was at 85.6 per cent and August at 88 per cent. Even if I assumed (a) 90 per cent revenue for September, October, November and December 2020 and (b) 95 per cent revenue for January, February and March 2021, total GST revenue for FY21 will still be some 17 per cent less than what it was in FY20, or a gross shortfall of 1 per cent of nominal GDP.

My fear is that, confronted with such a large gap, the Finance Ministry may be tempted to put a larger number of goods and services into the 18 per cent and 28 per cent GST slabs. And that the revenue-starved GST Council might concur.

Other Challenges

One of the greatest challenges facing India today is the parlous situation of state finances. At the best of times, the states were running an aggregate fiscal deficit of 2.5 per cent to 3 per cent of GDP. COVID has made things worse—not only because of additional health-related expenditure and fall in revenues, but also because it has exposed serious shortcomings in public health infrastructure across most states. How this challenge will be met, and what role the union will have in financing this, is going to be an important determinant of a state's ability to offer health services to its citizens.

No less a challenge is banking. Credit growth of SCBs considerably weakened in the first half of FY20, deteriorated further in the second half and has remained seriously muted from April 2020 onwards. Deposits have grown at a much faster rate as enterprises and households have foregone expenditures in favour of savings. Faced with a sudden excess of liabilities, banks have perforce parked their additional deposits in relatively low-yield treasury bills.

Indeed, banks face worse prospects. The Supreme Court, which has made it a habit to deliver opinions on economic and financial matters, passed an interim order on 3 September 2020, saying that accounts not declared as NPAs as on 31 August shall not be so declared until further notice. It has further delayed matters by also hearing petitions demanding waiver of interest, and interest on interest, on the suspended equated monthly instalments (EMIs) during the moratorium period. Any adverse judgement on that account can further batter the finances of banks and non-banking finance companies. Moreover, there is a serious risk of many corporate lenders demanding that their repayment period be extended, depending on the recommendations of the RBI's newly formed K.V. Kamath Committee, and what the central bank accepts. In addition, there are the NPAs.

In a baseline scenario, gross NPAs are expected to burgeon from 8.5 per cent on 31 March 2020 to 12.5 per cent on 31 March 2021, and under a stress scenario, to 14.7 per cent. Unsurprisingly, the worst affected will be the public sector banks, where the gross NPA ratio is predicted to increase at the very least from 11.3 per cent in March 2020 to 15.2 per cent in March 2021—and to 16.3 per cent under very severe stress.[37] In such a situation, banks will be loath to lend, especially to small traders and medium- and small-scale enterprises, unless the exchequer agrees to cover a significantly greater part of the cost than what has been proposed by the finance minister.

Buoyed by good agricultural output, some commentators have claimed to see 'green shoots'. Unfortunately, the hard facts are that the exchequer is in tatters; banks, especially the state-owned ones, are under severe strain and need recapitalization for which the central government does not have the funds, and we have a

---

[37] For these and other details, see RBI, *Financial Stability Report* (July 2020), especially Chapter II.

scenario where much of the real economy provides no succour.

Of course, optimists would claim that here lies our one-time opportunity to drive real reforms. Faced with COVID and the Chinese border threat, we can finally go the whole hog, such as knocking off all small-scale industry reservations, boosting defence production, focusing on tariff reforms and export expansion, fashioning significant free trade agreements, significantly simplifying tax procedures, undertaking labour market and urban land reforms, focusing on creating sound urban infrastructure, slum redevelopment and affordable low-income housing, creating more highways and better multi-modal logistics, accelerating banking reforms, privatizing state-owned enterprises and public sector banks, actively encouraging private investment, transforming public health and higher education, and creating the kind of governance that can sustain such reforms.

Each of these reforms has been emphasized time and again by many economists and pro-reform writers. Yet, it needs asking why is it that in the 29 years after July 1991, many have not seen the light of day? To me, it has everything to do with the political economy of reforms: of how the governing class—politicians and bureaucrats—view fundamental change.

The attitude of the former is to disagree if a reform doesn't benefit them. And of the latter is never to say 'no' to the political masters, and to convey that necessary action is being taken, when in fact none is. It helps that very few ministers have either the interest or gumption to challenge their civil servants and force them to do what is needed in a clear, time-bound manner. There are exceptions. But these have been few and far between.

Consider privatization. In 2016, PM Narendra Modi explicitly directed NITI Aayog to identify public sector enterprises for privatization. A detailed list was sent to his office, with the rationale for each privatization. The cabinet approved the list, which was then sent to the Department of Investment and Asset

Management for execution and monitoring. It has remained resolutely stuck there, without a single privatization. And this is a fairly simple reform.

Regrettably, therefore, I am no longer an optimist. Yes, I want these reforms. I want to claim that COVID gives us the opportunity as 1991 did. But I don't see these happening in any hurry. Not even under PM Modi, who is no less a 'statist' than Indira Gandhi.

So, I don't believe COVID will bring about fundamental path-breaking changes in the structure, rules and dynamism of the economy. I don't see the transformation of a lumbering elephant to a leaping tiger. But, in my more optimistic days, I occasionally see a marginally faster elephant—which is apposite for a nation that could have made it, but hasn't.

◆

Omkar Goswami is an economist and the chairman of CERG Advisory, a company that deals with economic advisories and corporate consultancy. He is an author of over 70 published papers and four books.

CENTRE–STATE LESSONS FROM THE CORONAVIRUS PANDEMIC

Indira Rajaraman

The points of entry into India of the novel coronavirus were limited in the first instance to a small number of international airports, and at the time of the first communication from the World Health Organization (WHO) dated 11 January 2020, potential entry of the virus was further limited to travellers entering the country from China. Kerala alone, among the states in India, was quick and effective in meeting the threat.

There was no standing Centre–state communication channel, whereby other states could have adopted the steps taken by Kerala to contain the spread of the virus. Such a channel could function as a continual multi-nodal public policy learning framework, whereby states in a federal entity can learn from one another.

The first press release on the novel coronavirus on 17 January 2020[38] from the Ministry of Health and Family Welfare (MoHFW) cites the 11 January 2020 WHO communication as having said that 'keeping in view the limited human-to-human transmission, the risk at global level is perceived to be low'. The WHO clearly failed to perceive the high risk posed by the new pathogen. However, 'as a matter of abundant precaution the Ministry of

---

[38]Ministry of Health and Family Welfare. (2020, January 17). 'Health Ministry reviews preparedness for Novel Corona Virus(nCoV)'. Accessed at: https://pib.gov.in/PressReleseDetail.aspx?PRID=1599665

Health has instructed screening of international travellers from China at designated airports namely, Delhi, Mumbai and Kolkata through thermal scanners'.

Another press release[39] the same day issued a travel advisory for visitors returning to India from China, in spite of the WHO's risk assessment that 'the mode of transmission is unclear', and 'there is little evidence of significant human-to-human transmission'. The advisory was for travellers returning from China to voluntarily self-declare at the airport if they feel sick upon arrival, or within a month of their return.

A later press release of 20 January 2020[40] extended thermal screening to four additional airports at Chennai, Bengaluru, Hyderabad and Kochi. This is the earliest date on which an airport falling in Kerala was included within the ambit of the MoHFW warning system. Subsequent MoHFW press releases dated 22 January[41] and 23 January[42] merely report the number of flights and passengers screened, but no detected cases; another dated 25 January[43] announced extension of thermal screening to 12 additional airports in addition to the previous seven.

The important point to note is that even by 25 January, there was no advice from the MoHFW going beyond thermal screening at designated airports, and advising voluntary self-reporting by passengers a month after return.

---

[39]Ministry of Health and Family Welfare. (2020, January 17). 'Novel coronavirus outbreak in China: Travel advisory to travelers visiting China'. Accessed at: https://pib.gov.in/PressReleseDetail.aspx?PRID=1599666

[40]Ministry of Health and Family Welfare. (2020, January 20). 'Outbreak of Novel Coronavirus in China: Actions taken by the Health Ministry'. Accessed at: https://pib.gov.in/PressReleseDetail.aspx?PRID=1599901

[41]Ministry of Health and Family Welfare. (2020, January 22). '9156 Passengers from 43 Flights screened for novel Coronavirus (nCoV); No case of nCoV has been detected'. Accessed at: https://pib.gov.in/PressReleseDetail.aspx?PRID=1600137

[42]Ibid.

[43]Ibid.

The Kerala Guidelines

It was at that point that Kerala went beyond the national advisory to issue guidelines applicable within the state jurisdiction, of which an updated version dated 26 January is available in the public domain.[44] Running into 27 pages of impressive detail, it has the following provisions for asymptomatic passengers arriving from notified countries, where the list was to be continually updated.

Section 3, Page 5:

> (4) Names of asymptomatic passengers from said origins will be forwarded by Airport Health Officer/Ports Health Officer to SSO IDSP-ADHS PH [State Surveillance Officer of the Integrated Disease Surveillance Programme-Additional Director of Health Services, Primary Health] Kerala and State Nodal Officer Dr Amar S. Fettle which will also be shared to the DSO/DSU [District Surveillance Officer/District Surveillance Unit] of the concerned district.
>
> (5) These passengers will have to be kept under close surveillance under home quarantine by the concerned DSO/PHC [primary health centre] Medical officer [MO] for 28 days from the time of departure from the affected country or from the time of contact with a suspected/confirmed patient.
>
> (7) Provision for passengers arriving by land transport from other airports like Bangalore, to be identified at community level through the same network.

Section 8, Page 11:

> Daily monitoring coordinated by PHC MO on information received from DMO [district medical officer]/DSO, and by

---

[44]https://dhs.kerala.gov.in/wp-content/uploads/2020/03/ncorona_26012020.pdf; accessed 14 July 2020.

the designated area field staff.

Referral and transportation management if indicated by development of symptoms, under direct liaison between DSO and PHC MO.

The Kerala provisions for surveillance, quarantining and daily monitoring of asymptomatic arriving passengers went well beyond the national instructions for voluntary self-reporting as issued by the MoHFW. The formal instructions were to forward names of asymptomatic passengers to the SSO IDSP, a nationwide MoHFW initiative, and to the DSU of the concerned district where the destination of the arriving passenger lay.

Here is a clear example of how a subnational state in a federal structure was activating a nationally instituted decentralized reporting structure, which was being completely disregarded in the national instructions issued by MoHFW to all states. Surveillance was also extended, using the same network, to identify passengers having arrived from infected countries at airports outside Kerala from the notified points of origin, and arriving in the state by land transportation.

There is clear evidence of integration within Kerala between the surveillance structure of the nationwide IDSP and the state-level primary health vertical, since responsibility for daily monitoring of home quarantine was placed under the direct supervision of the PHC MO, using designated area field staff.

The final and most noteworthy feature is the provision for referral and transportation of those under surveillance, who developed symptoms, to care facilities.

Altogether, these instructions are outstanding in terms of last-mile coverage, closing all loopholes, ensuring no possible avenue of infection was left uncovered and that those infected were cared for towards full recovery.

Although the Kerala guidelines document was displayed online and therefore accessible to all, it seems not to have been noticed by the MoHFW or the IDSP. Cognisance of such state initiatives would have been facilitated if there had been a Centre–state portal, where Kerala could have posted its guidelines, and further reported infection rates among asymptomatic passengers quarantined and followed up after arrival.

Integrated Disease Surveillance Programme

The IDSP website states its mission as the establishment of 'a decentralised State-based surveillance system for epidemic prone diseases to detect the early warning signals so that timely and effective public health actions can be initiated in response'. It proudly reports that 90 per cent of districts are directly reporting weekly disease surveillance data on the portal. These figures would have been routinely reported from Kerala in the weeks following the guidelines, but in the absence of any underlying information on the initiatives undertaken in that state towards better identification, would have merely been taken as evidence of the rapid spread of the disease in Kerala (as indeed did happen).

The reporting structure presupposes that decision-making and initiatives will be confined to the Centre, with states merely assigned the role of reporters from the field in prescribed formats. There is no provision for reporting of state-level initiatives and their outcomes, so that information can be laterally disseminated, for direct emulation by states without having to wait for national directives.

The IDSP was started with World Bank's assistance in 2004, but shifted later to domestic funding and at some point folded into the National Health Mission (NHM),[45] a national scheme

---

[45]The IDSP is an insignificant component of the total flow, typically 0.2–0.3 per cent of total NHM funds.

with co-funding by states in prescribed shares. Starting from the horizon of the 14th Finance Commission in FY16, the state share was raised from the previous level of 25 per cent to 40 per cent, and the central share correspondingly reduced from 75 per cent to 60 per cent.[46]

The IDSP is part of an NHM component called 'flexible pool for communicable diseases [FPCD]'. Far from enabling flexible or rapid responses in the field, the rigid structure governing NHM fund flows seems designed to ensure failure to respond. The deficiencies of that structure were exposed in the only detailed study of the flow of NHM funds in a paper titled 'Utilisation, Fund Flows and Public Financial Management under the National Health Mission'.[47] The paper has an in-depth focus on three states, Bihar, Maharashtra and Odisha, for two years FY16 and FY17, yielding six data points in all.

NHM funds are segregated by component. Even within the FPCD, there are separate components for each disease, such as tuberculosis or leprosy, and funds for each component are released separately, at times not known in advance.[48] Separate accounts by component have to be maintained by the ultimate receiving agency in the states, the state health societies (SHSs), and by the further downstream district-level sub-offices of the SHSs. This deflects attention towards maintenance of records rather than towards addressing the burden of communicable diseases.

---

[46]This was a consequence of the raising of the statutory unconditional share of states in the Centre's tax revenues from 32 per cent to 42 per cent starting with year FY16, as recommended by the 14th Finance Commission for FY16 to FY20 quinquennium, further extended by the 15th Finance Commission to FY21 and adjusted down to 41 per cent because of one state having been split into two union territories.

[47]Mita Choudhury and Ranjan Kumar Mohanty. (2019). 'Utilisation, Fund Flows and Public Financial Management under the National Health Mission', *Economic and Political Weekly*, LVI: 8 (23 February); pp. 49–57

[48]Not even uniform across states.

Issue of sanction orders at the Centre for fund transfer varies in timing by NHM component. The data points in the Chaudhury–Mohanty paper show that sanctions were issued well beyond the start of the fiscal year, although the delays might have become shorter since then.[49]

The IDSP, in five of the six data points in the Choudhury–Mohanty paper, was sanctioned for release at the Centre between November and February, a few months before the end of the fiscal year. This was for a programme to enable public health responses to the early warning signals of an epidemic.

Clearly, a system of this kind presupposes that the funds issued in a fiscal year will be partially unutilized and be available for use in the early months of the next fiscal year.[50] Unutilized funds with the SHSs are formally included in the budgetary allocation for the next fiscal year.[51] However, the further problem with calling this unutilized is that the budgetary allocation may not have been fully released. This may be particularly true of the state contribution of 40 per cent, which may be only fractionally fulfilled, and in proportions varying across components.

A further delay in fund transmission was added at the start of FY15, when NHM funds had to be routed through state treasuries,

---

[49] On account of the advancement of the date of presentation of the central budget to two months before the start of the fiscal year starting with FY18, these sanction delays might have become shorter. In the paper, for the six data points, the major component was sanctioned typically six months after the start of the fiscal year, towards end-September. The earliest for any component was end-June. Sanctions for other small components were dribbled out after September, and went into March, the last month of the fiscal year.

[50] The utilization ratio of central funds allocated for the FPDC component, into which IDSP is folded, is not surprisingly a mere 55 per cent on average across all states in the country.

[51] However, there is a puzzle here. If that were the case, the quarterly pattern of expenditure should be evened out. That does not seem to be the case in the Choudhury–Mohanty study.

instead of being directly released to the SHSs as in previous years,[52] a change paradoxically recommended by a committee appointed in 2010 to improve accountability.[53] The number of approvals required, and thus the time taken, for fund release from state treasury to SHS, varied widely between the three states studied in the Choudhury–Mohanty paper, from three months or more (Bihar), to a little over two months (Maharashtra), to a month or less (Odisha).

Maintenance of continuity in any component of health delivery is seriously challenged in the face of a funding process, with the kind of uncertainties and delays detailed above. Despite the availability of the unutilized overhang at the start of the fiscal year, there would be funding shortages for particular components at various points in time during the year, co-existing with underutilization in other components. At such times, they are reported to prioritize disbursement not by programme so much as by budget head, with salaries given first priority.

It is not clear whether the SSO and DSO posts under the IDSP are fully funded under the NHM or are functions grafted onto state and district officers in the state's own health vertical. If the latter, the surveillance programme is likely to run more smoothly than if they are posts funded by the NHM, whose funding can be best described as fitful. Much of the IDSP funding probably goes towards the training of data entry operators and computer equipment within the state. Since these elements of non-salary expenditure are low-priority items, the functioning of the reporting system cannot possibly be very effective.

The final element in this numbingly defeatist structure is the further delay in release of funds from the SHSs to the district-

---

[52]Part of a general change across all centrally sponsored schemes, which are co-funded with states.
[53]The committee was chaired by C. Rangarajan. The members were Nitin Desai, Ravinder Dholakia, M.G. Rao and D.K. Srivastava.

level end-use point, which is where health expenditures actually need to happen. This is where the Kerala system of integrating the state's own health vertical, primed by the state's own fiscal resources, with the externally funded surveillance overlay enabled it to prove so effective.

Corona Outcomes in Kerala

As already mentioned, the Kerala initiative would have shown a higher case load count in the months before the lockdown, since it was far ahead of the rest of the country in identifying cases arriving through international airports. Chart 1 below shows the daily growth rate in Kerala and the rest of the country from the beginning of the first lockdown on 25 March 2020 upto 15 July 2020, which was a month and a half after the end of the successive lockdowns. The first lockdown brought the Kerala rate down to near zero since prior case arrivals were already identified, unlike the rest of the country, which continued to record new cases transmitted by prior case arrivals.

The Kerala daily growth rate ramped up in mid-May to equivalence with the national rate at around the 5 per cent mark. The reason for this was the huge influx of returning non-resident Indians (NRIs) into Kerala, principally from the Gulf, starting with the first flight on 7 May under Phase 1 of the Vande Bharat Mission. Under Phase 1, which went on until 17 May, 17 out of a total of 84 flights were destined for Kerala airports alone (Kochi, Kozhikode, Kannur and Trivandrum), carrying a total of nearly 4,000 passengers. The pressure of passengers arriving from overseas got stepped up rapidly with Phase 2 running from 19 May to 23 June, with a total of 578 flights landing in Indian airports.[54] Aggregating across the five phases, there were a total

---

[54]The source of data on Vande Bharat missions to fly home NRIs from overseas

of 3,305 flights into India. For states like Kerala, these incoming flights marked an abrupt end, starting 7 May to the domestic lockdowns, with a daily influx of passengers from some of the most afflicted countries in the world. However, because of the initial advantage, the share of Kerala in total national cases remained low all through the period (Chart 2).

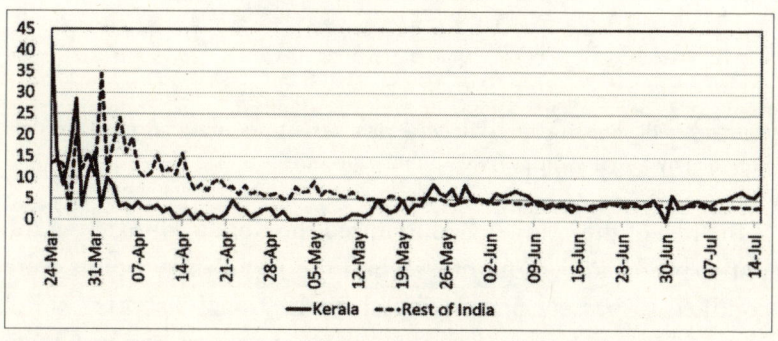

Chart 1: Daily % growth rate of corona cases
24 March to 15 July 2020

Source: Credit Suisse daily state-wise data series, assembled from daily data provided by MoHFW https://www.mohfw.gov.in/

Notes: The national lockdown markers are (1:25 March to 13 April); (2: 14 April to 3 May); (3: 4–17 May); (4: 18–31 May). This was followed by three numbered unlock periods, covering the months of June, July and August, respectively. The first influx of air passengers began during Lockdown 3 with the first Vande Bharat flight from UAE to Kerala on 7 May, and continued steadily thereafter (see text). The lagged impact in Kerala is visible from the middle of May, and was more pertinent than the end of the lockdowns on the case growth rates.

---

locations is https://www.mea.gov.in/vande-bharat-mission-list-of-flights.htm, accessed on 12 August 2020. The flights were grouped into five phases, Phase 1 (7–17 May, 84 flights); Phase 2 (19 May–23 June, 578 flights); Phase 3 (23 June–2 July, 553 flights); Phase 4 (3 July–1 August, 1,082 flights); and Phase 5 (1–30 August, 1,008 flights).

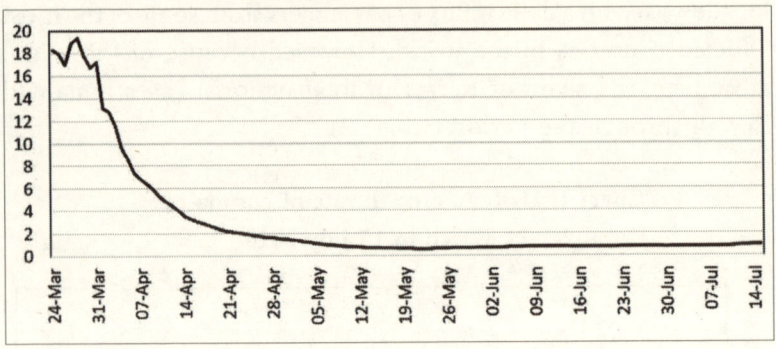

Chart 2: Kerala % share of national total cases 24 March to 15 July 2020

Source: Credit Suisse daily state-wise data series, assembled from daily data provided by MoHFW https://www.mohfw.gov.in/

If the rest of the country had followed the Kerala approach in the initial pre-lockdown months, when the virus entry points were confined to passengers arriving at international airports, and at least in January to passengers arriving from China, the lockdown would have brought the growth rate down to near-zero (as it did in Kerala), and post-lockdown, would have grown again with the fresh influx starting 7 May with the Vande Bharat flights, but from a lower base.

Since with free borders, no single state can keep its case growth rate appreciably below the national level, it is only the case fatality rate that can truly test the effectiveness of the Kerala model, which was not about case identification alone, but about arranging for referral and transportation to care centres for those identified. Fatality rates as a per cent of concurrent cases are shown in Chart 3. Deaths as a concurrent per cent of cases when cases are growing in number will be lower than as a per cent of cases at the point of diagnosis, but that bias affects both series, as shown in Chart 3. The Kerala fatality rates are well below the 1 per cent mark; the rest of India is at an average of 3 per cent.

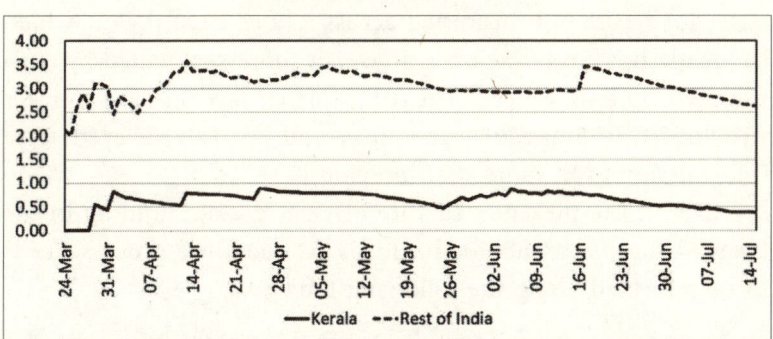

Chart 3: Fatality rates as a % of concurrent cases
24 March to 15 July 2020

Source: Credit Suisse daily state-wise data series, assembled from daily data provided by MoHFW https://www.mohfw.gov.in/

Conclusion

The response of Kerala to the initial entry of the COVID pandemic in terms of immediate identification of those infected and arrangements for cure of the identified are shown in this chapter, along with the outcomes in terms of case share and fatality rates relative to the rest of the country. The progress made by the state was set back starting mid-May due to the opening up of airports to bring back migrants from the Gulf and other points of origin, which raised the case growth rate to equivalence with that in the rest of India.

Outbreaks of communicable diseases call for immediacy of response. There has to be an open portal for continuing communication across states whereby improved processes and responses can be adopted, along the lines of the yardstick competition model, which is one of the proclaimed advantages of a federal structure of governance. Had that been in place, the pandemic could have been nipped in the bud when its entry points were limited to a few international airports.

The larger failure in health outcomes in India is embedded in structural problems with fund flows. The Centre's funding to states for health is transmitted across a huge trust divide, which has made the fund flow over time ever more segmented by end-use prescriptions. Since April 2014, further layers in the transfer structure have impeded fund flow, and so have delayed fund transmission even more than previously.

Even if the present structure of Centre–state funding in the form of specific grants for health is retained, the process needs to be reformed along the following four lines:

- Merging components, so that the flexible pool for communicable diseases is truly flexible and not segmented into separate components for specific diseases, such as tuberculosis. The total NHM flow should be divided into at most four components, with flexibility of use within each.
- The calendar for sanction orders at the Centre should be known in advance, and adhered to within a margin of +/- two working days.
- States should be required to streamline the administrative process for release of NHM funds (which, after April 2014, flow to the state treasury in the first instance), such that the SHS, the agency charged with execution, receives funds no later than 10 days after receipt at the state treasury. The time and attention of state government functionaries used up in shepherding the approval process for fund release from the state treasury is a deadweight loss that no state government can afford.
- The mandatory contribution of 40 per cent by states is worked into the budgetary allocation, but not always fully released in practice. The low utilization rates worked out on a denominator of allocations reflect this phenomenon

in part. This can be rectified by requiring states to commit their contribution to the NHM budget in absolute terms rather than as a per cent of the total, in amounts that they feel confident they can deliver.

In conclusion, it must be pointed out that the process failures, which have crippled health outcomes in the country, are not specific to any political party or ideology. They are quite simply an outcome of the fact that processes underlying fund flow have not been paid the attention they deserve. As the COVID pandemic has shown, a failure on the health front is not only tragic in itself, but could defeat the larger economic ambitions of the country.

◆

Indira Rajaraman was a member of the Thirteenth Finance Commission. From 1994 until her retirement in 2007, she held the Reserve Bank of India Chair at the National Institute of Public Finance and Policy, Delhi, and from 1976 to 1994 she was on the Economics faculty of the Indian Institute of Management, Bangalore. She was a visiting scholar at Harvard and Stanford Universities (1984–85), and at the Fiscal Affairs Department of the International Monetary Fund (2004).

Note: This article earlier appeared as 'Centre-state lessons from the Corona Virus pandemic' in Indian Federalism Perspectives, 1(2), 2000 (September).

PANDEMIC AND THE PEOPLE

TOWARDS A PEOPLE-CENTRED POST-COVID POLICY

Rama Bijapurkar

COVID-19 has held up a mirror to India's 'people reality', forcing us to take cognisance of the human face of our economy. The big message from the pandemic and lockdown experience is that policy is all about people, especially the poorer half of India. The experience has necessitated that we take a closer look at the 'people consequences' of policy than we have in recent times.

An even more sobering lesson is what we learnt as we looked across the world to see what policies were being implemented to deal with the situation—that policy choices are totally intertwined with the values and priorities of a society or a nation. In the US, the Mecca of individualism, the debate was between laws to curb the spread and the rights of the individual, including whether being forced to wear a mask in public was a violation of the fundamental rights of a person. (In India, the government fines us if we don't wear one.) Some countries in Europe thought that putting their elderly at risk was inevitable and acceptable for the larger economic stability of the country. In Britain, there's a battle over whether or not children should be at school. China dealt with it with little room for debate.

Choices made by policymakers and policy recipients around the world provide a most interesting window through which to view how the values and priorities of a society drive policy.

It also shows us that there can't be a global best practice and each country has to study what others are doing but act in accordance with its own values. In India, our choice has been lives vs. livelihood, and the needle of choice has settled on the 'lives' side; people have accepted the nanny state. TikTok, which I dearly miss, was the best place to see the mood of the 'aam junta' (common people). My favourite video was one where a young woman is getting ready to happily step out of the house and the PM's hologram appears saying, 'Get back in there or I will shut off your internet'. And she scurries back inside! All that pundits and commentators, even of impeccable academic pedigree, could say was, 'Please don't destroy livelihoods but also save lives!' There were no suggestions forthcoming on how to balance these two objectives. Even those who said 'choose livelihood' said that it was because the poor could not live if livelihoods were severely impaired.

COVID has forced us all to engage with the aam junta. How they earn, how they live, what choices they make, what they eat, their choices of lives vs. livelihood, and so on. And that engagement should stay with policymaking and policy advice going forward.

Hasn't the connection between people and policy always been the cornerstone of Indian public and economic policy? The first step in our post-COVID policy thinking is to honestly ask ourselves if this connection has indeed been so, particularly in the past two decades. My answer is that the link has weakened and we need to course correct.

In the pre-COVID world, policymakers and business leaders built their mental models of India in terms of wonderful macro numbers or benign-sounding conceptual constructs, pushing into the dim background the human states of being that underlie these. They have embraced good macro numbers, such as total GDP, and sidestepped bad ones, such as per capita GDP, in case of the poorer half of Indians. They have also used constructs, such as 'demographic dividend' (and ideas, such as 'demographic destiny'), which extol age demographics and ignore the poor education level of the youth. The macro and aggregate view of India is indeed wonderful. Thinking of India merely as a GDP number or growth number, or in terms of a world GDP ranking number, makes everything smell of roses.

Constructs such as 'informal sector' sound a lot less threatening than 'daily wage earner' or 'hawker'. When we say workers, one usually thinks of those in factories, maybe with no 'permanent job', but with regular salaries. Similarly, 'demographic dividend' or even 'demographic disaster' is not as stark as saying only x per cent of young people have finished school. As India climbs world rankings, our dismal demographics seem even less important. Ten per cent penetration of anything in India makes it stack up very well in world rankings, given our large population. If we forget the way the number was derived, we forget that only 10 per cent penetration has been achieved and policy must work to make the other 90 per cent happen, and that it is too early to declare policy victory.

The same goes for the metric 'number of people lifted out of poverty'. It does not explain how they were lifted out of poverty (what was the nature of jobs) and what being 'lifted out of poverty' means. When the number game is played, then metrics or poverty lines are chosen, as befits the number. The underlying fundamentals of Indians' lives and livelihoods have not been taken much notice of except by the 'povertarianism' brigade, who saw only poverty, deprivation, wretchedness of spirit and a need for handouts as the policy prescription. They did not see or accept how poor Indians were thinking. They did not see the desire for opportunity, or for capability to have a shot at that opportunity. If the macro number celebrators saw rising GDP as an automatic signal of a better life for all, the 'povertarians' saw a policy of handouts as a means to do that. The former took the 'let them eat the cake' view of the common people of India. It's okay if you are only skilled enough to be a construction labourer, but you have a cell phone thanks to GDP growth (and China). The latter took the 'give them fish, what use do they have for a fishing rod?' view of the common people of India. The 'people view' of India puts them at the centre of policy design, not just at election time, and that view should drive policymaking going forward. This is not anti-market, nor is it populism. For lack of a better word it is people-ism or a people-centred policy.

Dismal Occupation Demographics Needs Urgent Attention

If there is just one thing that policy needs to address, it is the occupation profile of the aam junta.

Occupation Mainly Contributing to Household Income

Table 1

	Urban Mn. HH	Rural Mn. HH	Total Mn.	% of all HH
CASUAL LABOUR: Daily wage/piece rate (eg., construction, cleaning, loading, agricultural labour)	24	67	91	32
PETTY TRADER: Hawker/street vendor with no permanent establishment	6	5	11	4
INDIVIDUAL SERVICE PROVIDER: Those with varying degrees of skills (eg., plumber, electrician, dhobi, delivery person)	7	7	14	5

INFORMAL SALARIED WORKER: Workers with mostly no job contract, grade IV type (eg., peon, messenger, security guard, driver, office boy, household help, factory worker)	25	20	45	16
SHOP OWNER: Business owners with permanent retail establishments/registered stores (eg., contractor, wholesaler, kirana owner	15	11	26	9
SUPERVISORY/CLERICAL SALARIED WORKERS	4.5	1.7	6	2
SALARIED PROFESSIONALS: Self-employed professionals, officers/executives earning regular salary	4.4	3.4	8	3
PENSIONERS: Others who live off remittances, rent, welfare support	7.3	18	25	9
AGRICULTURISTS: Self-employed in farming	-	52	52	19
Total number of households	281 million			

Source: ICE 360° data from People Research on India's Consumer Economy[55]

Table 1 shows the number of families dependent mainly on each kind of occupation in rural and urban India. The answer is beyond sad—it is quite chilling. One-third of Indian families depend on casual labour for their earnings. Another 4 per cent are dependent on petty trader occupations, such as hawkers and street vendors,

---

[55] R. Bijapurkar. (2020, April 12). Experts Explain: Loss of income; ground-up assessment of recovery support to households. Retrieved November 10, 2020, from https://indianexpress.com/article/explained/an-expert-explains-ground-up-assessment-of-recovery-support-to-households-6357022/

with no permanent establishment. In fact, they have no right to even the place where they keep their 'thela' or their makeshift stack. It is not an uncommon sight to see them fleeing from the police or paying 'hafta' to them every now and then in the big cities. They earn between ₹8,000–10,000 per family per month and even this modest income is a daily wage, dependant on whether there's work available or not. In good economy years, work is guaranteed and incomes may be higher; but the fact remains that the largest occupation group in this country is that of people doing manual labour. Increasingly, we are seeing machines replace people. We need to assess the price point of labour at which this switchover will start getting accelerated.

Recently, the seawater next to my building in Mumbai was reclaimed as part of a coastal road project. It has a large private company as contractor, and an estimated expenditure of ₹12,000 crore. The work progressed at an extraordinary speed, and what was most unusual about it was how little physical labour it utilized. At any point there were maybe three or four people on the site, probably supervisors; and upwards of 20 trucks, a few earth-moving equipment and a crane, which were doing all the work. We also know that even large investments in manufacturing are creating hardly transpose any jobs. So, the question is what do we do for the casual labourers and street-sellers on whom these 100 million families of India's 281 million families depend? The education level is also dismal in this group. Where does one begin to retrain and reskill the current members and future recruits to this group?

The skilling programmes of the government have typically picked company chieftains to lead them, and asked them to run skill-development missions. Mostly, their prescriptions did not even recognize this group, leave alone address their needs. Can they be given some sort of skill to make them join the ranks of the 5 per cent solo service providers? Since self-driving trucks are still a distant possibility in India, and there is a shortage of drivers, which threatens to impair the truck industry and is the bane of logistics business, can some be upgraded to drivers? Can they be upgraded to healthcare providers (low-end nursing)? Can they be trained to join the police force, given the poor police-to-population ratio that exists? Where are the other demand–supply gaps that can be plugged for people who are doing casual labour? What is the logical upward progression for them?

The topic of skilling is a highly debated one. But if the discussion can be shifted from grand strategies for mass skilling in a supply-sided manner to what can be done with over 100 million people engaged in casual labour, whose lot has not improved despite all the macro numbers, we may make some people-centred policies and have some real impact. This is not the domain of private corporates but of the government, and policy efforts on this have been few and far between.

If we could reverse the size of casual labour-dependant families and solo service provider-dependant (more skilled than casual labour) families, then we would have made real progress. Aggregator platforms, which are bound to grow in number and scale, and range from hyperlocal to pan-Indian, will then give them the next level of training, skill-upgradation and income.

Macro analysts say that if women joined the workforce, then the GDP would rise by some x per cent. This begs the question 'Join the workforce and do what?' A large chunk of 45 million families are dependent on informal grade IV-type service work, such as domestic helps and security guards in offices or in factories for unskilled work. Though they earn a regular salary, which is a better state to be in than daily wages, their jobs have no minimum wage, no health insurance, no day off in the week; they are subject to hire and fire. Policy pundits should examine whether imposing minimum wage for this group will help their cause or decrease demand for them. The answer will vary by sub-segment (nature of work) and geography. They should also examine whether there is any other way to help, such as unemployment and health insurance products that can be made available to them at an affordable price.

The other large chunk is households depending on agriculture or agriculture entrepreneurs. After the passage of the Farm Bills 2020, special efforts to enable this group to take advantage of the new avenues of opportunity will be initially needed. We can decide to leave this to the market and review it five years from now, while continuing to offer a package of subsidies until the small farmers' businesses become structurally more profitable.

This data also reiterates exactly how small the formally employed group is. Only 5 per cent families are dependent on formal sources of income. Can policies not focus excessively on them? A people-centred policy has to answer the question 'How will we improve this "people picture" of the fifth largest economy in the world that we pride ourselves to be?'

If there's one thing that we need to do post-COVID, it is to accept and address the occupation issue in a granular fashion. The surprise that most people claimed to have experienced at the number of migrant workers who had to leave their workplaces and trek home would not have been so great had we had a more people-centred view of Indians' occupations. The instability of their jobs and their fragile living conditions would have been clearer right from the start. In cities like Mumbai, for example in several bastis (slums), there is a shift system of housing that operates with night shift and day shift workers. But when none of them have any work, there is no place to live. Many of them have no cooking facilities and rely on outside vendors for food. During the lockdown, sources of food dried up, which was one of the many reasons for the mass migration.

It is really necessary to know, in a people-centred way, how Indians earn, spend, live and think, in order for policymakers to have the appropriate mental models of the ones they are designing policy for.

A People-centred View of Consumption

Consumption, to most policy thinkers and advisors, is the macro number of 'C' in the 'C + I + G' equation and one of the major components of GDP. The mental model of consumption is not a group of people who earn in different ways and make spending choices based on their earnings and their confidence levels. To businesses, consumption is a macro number called 'consumption expenditure', which is somehow created by macro forces. And like a tide that comes in (when PFCE grows) or goes out (when PFCE doesn't grow), it determines their business growth.

The question often asked by media and business leaders in times of slowing GDP growth is whether consumption will save the day. The mental model seems to be that PFCE and investment are separate macro indicators, whereas a people-centric view shows the connection between them clearly, especially given the Indian occupation structure. A sluggish investment environment in India means slow economic activity, and given the small number with regular salaried jobs, it does mean an immediate fall in income across the board and less money to spend on consumption. This is even more so given the very high rates of interest for personal loans for the kind of occupation that most people in India have. The high rates of interest, in turn, are because of the risks that such occupation profiles carry.

Knowing how much of consumption is accounted for by which occupation group in which part of India will help in understanding consumption slowdown better and prepare policy responses in a more targeted way, enabling businesses to see top-line risks better. Not all environmental bumps affect all parts of the consumption story equally.

Table 2 is our best estimate of how much of India's household consumption comes from which segment of people. Rural India accounts for over half of India's household consumption and the poorest 40 per cent of rural households account for almost 30 per cent of that, the same size as the so-called urban middle class, which is the richest 20 per cent of urban India. Casual labour accounts for a large chunk of consumption—almost 30 per cent of rural consumption and almost 20 per cent of urban consumption. Unless we change how Indians earn, we cannot bank on their consumption expenditure.

Table 2

Risk map of India's household consumption behaviour

Rural households account for 57% of all India household consumption expenditure while urban household consumption accounts for 43% of total consumption.

■ Totally at risk ■ Partially at risk ■ Relatively safe

RURAL CONSUMPTION

Row	Main occupation source of household income (% share of total rural household expenditure)	Poorest 40%	Middle 40%	Richest 20%	Overall rural
1	Farming and allied agriculture business	7.5	13.6	9.2	30
2	Non-farm micro business owners, individual service providers, petty traders, small shop owners	2.5	5.0	6.1	14
3	Salaried job (bank, govt, school teacher, company), self-employed professionals (doctor, lawyer, accountant)	1.6	5.9	10.6	18
4	Casual labour of all kinds	15.3	13.8	-	29
5	Other sources (remittances, pensions)	2.0	3.0	3.9	9
6	Total	29	41	31	100

URBAN CONSUMPTION

Row	Main occupation source of household income (% share of total urban household expenditure)	Poorest 40%	Middle 40%	Richest 20%	Overall urban
1	Salaried people and self employed professionals	6.3	17.1	19.4	43
2	Petty trader/shop vendor/individual service provider/shop owner/businessmen	7.2	12.7	9.1	29
3	Casual labour	8.2	9.5		18
4	Live on agriculture income	1	1.5	1.2	4
5	Live on rent, investments remittances from abroad etc.	1	2	2.6	6
6	Total	24	43	33	100

Source: Rama Bijapurkar and Dr Rajesh Shukla. (2020, April 20). Live Mint.

Understanding income and expenditure better will also help answer whether stimulating consumption will help the economy or not. The battle cry of 'let's stimulate consumption' is a popular one every time the economy is seen to be slowing down. A people-centred understanding of consumption will show two things. One, metrics like car sales are useless indicators of consumption slowdowns across the board because penetration of cars is really restricted to the top 20 per cent and far from saturation even there. It would also show the need to make the distinction between Ola/Uber/tourism 'investment' purchases of cars and household purchases of cars. It would also show us which segment of the population living where buys what and the extent to which their income has been affected due to any environmental shocks.

This will enable better policy responses rather than a rattling of the usual levers, some of which may not even be relevant for the situation or the segments affected. Further, a real people-centred understanding of consumption in India will show that Indians of all hues are very keen to consume. It's the income that they lack—the spirit is willing but the flesh is weak. Therefore, incentivizing them to spend isn't really necessary. Consumer confidence is nothing more than a derivative of income expectations. It is time to recognize that a weak desire to invest is not due to a lack of faith in the consumer story. Rather, it is a consequence of income expectations.

Weak investment is also due to a lack of faith in stability regulation and a peevish response to new norms of governance, bankruptcy-like situations of erstwhile big companies, Supreme Court rulings on sectors such as construction and telecom and so on. Therefore, the 'stimulate consumption' policy card cannot fix the totally different problem of supply-side constraints imposed by policy interventions.

Replacing China: How to Make It Possible

A lot of Indian households' well-being and quality of living has been on account of a plentiful flow of Chinese goods at exactly the price and performance points that the bottom half of Indian households (by income) require—saris, blankets, children's clothes, footwear and a range of necessities. These are households that many organized sectors, and large and established companies do not serve—they neither have the physical capacity nor the appetite to design such businesses and scale them. Why bother with low-margin, high-volume business when the opposite works quite well, more so when COVID damage to the top half is less compared to the bottom half.

Now with goods from China likely to dry up and with good reason, large swathes of Indians will not be able to buy substitutes at comparable price points. Consumption is not just a feel-good activity. It solves problems and adds value to the basic quality of living. Incentivizing and creating supply at that scale and with these price and performance characteristics will be a stretch for the weakened big firms of India Inc.

Large companies do not have the appetite to invest, and small companies cannot scale even if they had the money to invest. Policy should incentivize large companies, based on the unit price of items they sell, to start manufacturing for the mass market so that at least a handful of Chinese substitutes can come into being—incentivize in terms of interest rates and tax benefits. Maybe introduce another GST slab for mass market goods? At least it's for a worthwhile cause.

Holding the Price Line on Telecom

Cheap telecom rates have helped keep the beleaguered, modest-income Indian emotionally sane despite all the body blows that have come their way recently. A domestic helper who came to Mumbai leaving his family in Uttar Pradesh and got stuck here due to the lockdown could not go for his father's funeral but was able to watch it virtually. The cell phone is also India's number one productivity tool for, and aid to, family and social connectivity for the affiliative society that we are. It is also a major source of entertainment.

Keeping telecom rates low while preserving the competitive health of the sector constitutes the policy challenge. There's currently no employment in manufacturing, and if Indians are doomed to self-employment, then this is a must-have income and productivity booster irrespective of income.

Incentivizing Service Aggregator Platforms to Scale

If solo service will employ a large number of Indians and where the focus of skilling should be, aggregators for services that offer better benefits to the consumer and higher price realizations are the way to go. Such platforms do have to incur a fair amount of cost and effort in training though. Incentives in terms of lower interest rates and/or tax benefits for aggregators above a certain scale will encourage them to build scale. The IT industry has benefitted for decades from a tax holiday. It's time for the same ploy for service aggregators.

Keep Public Sector Banks and Financial Institutions Alive and Well

It is important to consider the overwhelming market share of public sector banks, especially amongst the poorest 40 per cent of India. Private banks do not want such customers. DBT systems and digital payment systems have been stress tested during COVID times and have delivered very well according to our data. While the push in policy circles is to privatize banks, we have not yet seen whether small finance banks fulfil their mission as they scale to serve modest-income consumers. Even in the payment space, Unified Payments Interface (UPI), the intel inside of interoperable payments, is not the creation of the private sector. Who private sectors serve is a people-centred input, which must be considered during policymaking on this count. In the healthcare sector, COVID has given us enough evidence and food for thought on how the market really works for modest-income consumers.

Conclusion

India is a large economy made up of lots and lots of small businesses and low-income consumers—truly the land of Lilliput. The overwhelming majority has very fragile sources of earning and low resilience to economic shocks. Our COVID experience has underscored the fragility of our macro numbers. Policymaking should recognize this and be designed for outcomes that strengthen the people and not declare policy victory based on large macro numbers as they have tended to ever since India entered the 'top 10' ranking of countries by GDP.

◆

Rama Bijapurkar is a recognized thought leader on market strategy and consumer behaviour. She is the co-founder of People Research on India's Consumer Economy and Citizen Environment, whose mission it is to provide a people-level view of India. She is also a professor of Management Practice at the Indian Institute of Management, Ahmedabad, and is on the governing board of the Centre for Policy Research, New Delhi.

BUILDING SAFETY NETS AND STORM SHELTERS

Meghnad Desai

The coronavirus pandemic has had a devastating effect on most economies around the world. The old debate about state vs. market has rumbled on, but many developing countries never trusted the market. The pandemic proved two things. Yes, in a pandemic, like in a war, you need the state rather than the market. Secondly, almost everywhere, the state has miserably failed to deal with the challenge. It does not matter whether the economy is developed, emerging or developing. Everyone has realized that they underinvested in public health, faced shortage of vital healthcare facilities, overburdened the system, piling suffering on people with comorbidities, and finally have arrived at a tasteless competition of numbers of dead per cases/capita.

Any investigation of mortality anywhere shows that the poor die disproportionately. They may be called Black and ethnic minorities in the UK and the US, or migrant labourers in India. But the surprise is that anyone is surprised. Development has not been an equalizing process. The last 25 years of globalization may have reduced the number of poor by the World Bank's definition, but up to 25 per cent of the population in every country has proved disproportionately susceptible to COVID due to a low and precarious economic status. Each nation can find one or more nation(s) below them in some statistic and become smug.

But we are all in this together, living a global failure.

The pandemic was a pure black swan, an unanticipated shock. It had no economic causes. At best, you can blame globalization and speedy international travel for the spread of the infection. But that apart, unlike in 2008 and the previous recessions, there was no endogenous economic reason for the pandemic. Never before have we had such a huge health shock to have been prepared for its economic costs. The Spanish flu of 1918 was after the war and there was a lot of dislocation in any case all over Europe.

Two further remarks are required about the economics of the coronavirus. One flatters economists and the other asks them to wake up. The flattering comment is that over the last few months, epidemiologists have proved no better than economists at either producing a convincing model of the origin and spread of infection nor have they been accurate in their forecasts. The two main coping strategies—mitigation (herd immunity) or suppression (lockdown)—have been tried with various degrees of hesitation, timidity and impatience by different countries, but there does not seem to be a significant difference between the mortality outcomes of the two strategies nor their economic cost. This is much like the forecasting models of economists.

I was brought up to believe that natural sciences were more solidly based on theory and experimental evidence, which grounded the models of scientists in reality. Well, that may be true of astrophysics but not of epidemiology. Banks are no longer permitted to use in-house models to assess their risk exposure, and have to subject them to examination by the Bank for International Settlements. We need an open window where epidemiological models can be scrutinized. When economists get it wrong, lives are not lost unlike when scientists get it wrong.

The wake-up call is to say that nothing in economics thus far modelled the fact of joint economic activity, be it consumption or production, in which proximity or distance was a significant variable. Coronavirus imposed special costs on contact-intensive activities. Thus, if consumption required company or face-to-face contact with the seller, social distancing made it difficult. Public transport was difficult but bicycles were fine. Economists may have to integrate proximity as a cost in their calculations.

Pre-COVID India

The Indian economy had been in a downward phase of the growth cycle since around the middle of 2016. On a longer trajectory, India had done well since 1991 but particularly well for 10 years, 1997–2007. The growth rate held up despite the Great Recession of September 2008. A GDP growth rate of high single digits became routine. Even since 2016, when growth had been slowing down, we were still thinking of 5 per cent as a low number. For an economy that seldom managed 5 per cent in its first 30 years, 1950–80, India seemed to have established a taller floor than before. Now I am not so sure, because by end of 2019–20 the GDP growth rate was down to 4.2 per cent. It is almost certain that 2020–21 is unlikely to yield a non-negative GDP growth rate. Preliminary estimates released recently showed that the economy had declined by 24 per cent in the first quarter of fiscal 2020–21. Projections for 2020–21 predict a 10–12 per cent negative growth in GDP. How far down it will go and how the bounceback will be shaped are open questions.

That said, I must add a slight worry. The Indian economy had a good 15 years after 1950, followed by low growth and famines for 25 years between 1965 and 1990. What followed were 25 years of a virtuously long cycle of high growth from 1991 to 2016. Has this cycle come to an end? Will India enter a long cycle of low growth? It is important to understand the growth cycle since 2016 to think of the post-COVID economy.

The reasons for the recent growth cycle were entirely monetary.

India has begun to behave like a developed economy, at least in its urban corporate sector. The credit market became rapidly dysfunctional with the NPAs of public sector banks becoming unsustainable, and then the non-banking credit sector hit a bad patch with the failure of Infrastructure Leasing & Financial Services (IL&FS). The initiation of the IBC was helpful, but the judicial process in the company law tribunal ran into problems and judicial delays lengthened. This meant that the effective cost of borrowing rose beyond the going rate of profitability. India was caught in a classic Wicksell–Hayek cycle caused by movements in expected rate of profitability relative to the cost of borrowing. When the cost of borrowing is raised because of rising risk for lenders, then the boom reverses into a downturn. The cure, however, lies not in manipulating the bank rate but restructuring banking, the credit market, the financial regulatory structure and the relevant judiciary structures, so that lending and borrowing can become healthy again. As it is now, recovering a debt is an expensive and time-consuming operation in India.

Recovery after COVID

The COVID pandemic has lasted longer than many countries expected. The possibility of a vaccine being available is high but its timing of arrival and being given to large populations are uncertain. It is safe to assume that the recovery would be unlikely to be V-shaped. The left, downward bit is here but the upward phase of the recovery may not come soon, nor be as sharp as a V shape indicates. Much of 2021 will be spent recovering. This may sound pessimistic but it is better to be cautious than assume that recovery will be either rapid or certain. Given that perspective, I wish to concentrate more on correcting longer-run structural weaknesses than hurry towards a return to business as usual.

Building Safety Nets

The coronavirus exposed the deep structural flaws of the Indian economy, like in an X-ray image. As it was, by July 2019, signs of demand slump were there. But what happened after the virus struck in February 2020 was enormous. Lockdown exposed a long-run structural fault in the Indian economy—the failure to absorb labour in productive employment. Successive plans since 1951 have failed to tackle the issue of surplus labour in both the rural and urban economy. Roughly speaking, there are 500 million male workers in the labour force. The LFPR of women (LFPR-W) is low, at around 20.8 per cent (as of late 2020), the lowest in Asia. That itself is a sign of lack of paid work opportunities. So, we are looking at 600 million employable workers plus another 400 million women at home.

Agriculture has 69 per cent self-employed and 44 per cent casual labour. Construction sector has 40 per cent of its labour force as casual.[56] COVID exposed 200 million workers, many of them migrants from distant states who had come to urban areas to work in the informal sector, to sudden and open unemployment. India has surplus labour in the rural areas as 60 per cent of the population lives there, but agriculture contributes only 16 per cent of GDP. Two-thirds of farmers are subsistence farmers relying on off-farm employment to supplement their incomes. These surplus workers can rely on MGNREGA each year as a cushion. The organized manufacturing sector has been capital-intensive and has stagnated, as indicated by its share of the GDP. Labour laws jealously protect workers in the small, organized sector. Contract labour has been hired in the organized sector but under precarious tenures. It is the informal sector in urban areas that has been absorbing surplus labour. The COVID pandemic has shown us

---

[56]RBI Annual Report cited in *Times of India*, 31 August 2020.

that at any time, up to half the labour force is either unemployed or underemployed.

The first 30 years built a public sector-owned manufacturing sector in the formal sector plus a bureaucracy well-cushioned from job or income insecurity. It was socialism for the few, and raw underdeveloped capitalism for the many.

Such income growth, as has taken place during the years before COVID, has been in the skilled service sector and organized manufacturing sector. These two sectors plus the middle and large farmers have generated high incomes. But they do not create new jobs. My guess is that the income growth-generating sectors account for around 100 million workers. The remaining 400–450 million are struggling.

Building a Welfare State

Before COVID, and even before the 2019 election, there were hopes of doubling India's GDP from $2.5 trillion to $5 trillion in five years. It was not feasible even then as it implied 14 per cent per-annum growth in GDP. Since India's real growth has never gone to double digits for any two years, it would require a healthy appreciation of the Indian rupee with respect to the US dollar to reach that goal. COVID makes the task even more difficult. India will start below $2 trillion at the end of 2020–21.

What COVID has shown is that India can throw up a welfare support structure rather quickly, which, while not a forethought, did work adequately. Here I am speaking of the income support schemes that were hastily devised and adapted for money to reach the people in need via DBT. Indeed the resilience of MGNREGA has been the one shiny spot during the crisis.

This resilience of the transfer mechanism is a structural strength of the Indian political economy. Through the 70-plus years of planning and economic policy, one of the successes has been government schemes to help the deprived sections. These schemes have attracted solid political support as well as turned out to be moderate enough to be fiscally affordable. (Compare persistent losses of public sector enterprises, especially banks or Air India, and you can put the money spent on entitlements in perspective.) COVID gives us the chance of coordinating these many schemes into a robust welfare structure. Indeed, the immediate short-term responses, such as the direct transfer of ₹500 to women's Jan Dhan accounts, have every merit of becoming permanent. As many as 20 crore women have received upwards of ₹30,000 crore. MGNREGA has benefited 4 crore households.

There has been some discussion of a Universal Basic Income (UBI). While I have been an advocate of UBI for the UK for a long time, it is difficult to install it in India, as people would not like to give up any of the existing benefits in exchange for UBI. There is also the political argument against UBI that undeserving people get it. There is, however, a case for extending a MGNREGA-type of scheme to urban informal sector workers. There should be an urban unemployment benefit of up to 100 days a year on the analogy of the rural scheme. I have been proposing this idea through the pandemic. Once surplus-labour households are covered in the rural as well as urban informal sectors, there will be a solid floor to the welfare state.

As far as UBI is concerned, I would favour a scheme that would be for women only. The transfer of ₹500 during the COVID crisis should be treated as a pilot scheme. The fact that the LFPR-W is low (the lowest in Asia) means that most women are doing unpaid work in the household. Indeed, even when women are at work for wages, they still have to do domestic work. So, UBI would be a great step forward for strengthening women's economic position. These three strands—MGNREGA, unemployment benefits for urban workers and a universal basic allowance for women—would be the floor of the welfare state.

What would help to further solidify this basic welfare package is the provision of affordable housing. In Mumbai, you see Bombay Development Directorate chawls in Worli, which were built for industrial workers of the earlier years of the twentieth century. Cheap but affordable urban housing on such a model would generate jobs while it is being constructed and allow urban workers, if unemployed, not to have to return to their rural roots as they had to with much misery during the pandemic.

During Modi 1.0, schemes were launched for health and pensions for many sections of the population. Ayushman Bharat covered the bottom third of the population. But COVID exposed the severe shortage of hospital facilities even in metros such as Delhi. Even in normal times, every public hospital is a scene of overcrowding, with families squatting on the grounds of hospitals or in corridors. While there is great support for building the All India Institute for Medical Sciences facilities around the country, what is needed is a network of small hospitals on the model of Delhi's mohalla clinics. There has been a tendency to extend rights to free healthcare without providing the supply of adequate infrastructure. This only makes the nominally free healthcare expensive in terms of time delays and lack of sufficient care due to shortage of staff and facilities. COVID has shown us not only the size of the need but also the overwhelming economic value of investing in public health. The key is to have many small but local health clinics on the lines of Delhi's mohalla clinics to provide immediate diagnosis and prescription or even overnight stay for patients with acute problems.

Income support, affordable housing and health service together will make a sturdy welfare state for the majority of Indians who have not benefited from 70 years of growth. It will repay because improvement in health, both physical and mental, will reduce costs of economic wastage, such as the one we saw across the country during the lockdown. It is also a dividend long overdue for the majority.

The Productive Economy

Between 1991 and 2016, India was doing many things right as far as the productive economy is concerned. The economy was opened up to trade and capital liberalization, and India doubtless benefited from the long boom of the new age of globalization. When the long boom ended in 2008, India faltered but recovered. It looked as if the high growth rate would continue. As I have hinted above, the growth-generating sector, the modern services sector, plus the infrastructure construction sector flourished through the 25-year virtual cycle. But eventually the pre-1991 structures in financial markets, such as nationalized banking and the mechanism for regulating the financial sector—inefficient but bureaucratic—proved inadequate. The market could have disciplined banks laden with bad debts. But state protection removed market discipline. Even private commercial banks misbehaved in such a system as the bankers learned to game the regulatory system. The spate of bad debts, the successful evasion of repayment of debts by crony capitalists and the slowness of realizing the problem meant that the introduction of IBC, while necessary, did not prove sufficient.

High growth rates will only be achieved by developing this modern sector. Agriculture is unlikely to grow at above 4 per cent as it is at present, though the removal of old restrictions on farmers' freedom to sell output will help. Perhaps the development of high value-added market gardening activities may change agriculture into a high-growth activity. It is not politically feasible but economically desirable to retire subsistence farmers, or at least persuade their younger generation to retire from cultivation, offer them local manufacturing jobs and release the land for more efficient use. These transformations will take a much longer perspective. A rural industrialization scheme of sufficient ambition can transform the rural areas. Instead of contributing one-sixth of GDP with three-fifths of the population, the rural economy could become prosperous by matching its economic contribution to its population size.

The biggest obstacle to such transformation is the fixed idea that farmers must be poor. An urban worker cannot hope to have his debts cancelled, but say the word 'kisaan' and the hearts of policymakers melt, and farmers' debts are forgiven. 'Friends of farmers' have ensured that their lands are impossible to sell, so they are not allowed to quit farming and so the farmers stay poor. They cannot prosper by giving up farming. The Land Acquisition Act 2013 is a monument to such paternalistic obstacles set by the Congress–UPA government. The incoming Modi government tried to change it but with no luck. Similar virtuous pauperization has been visited upon many tribal groups who live in areas with mineral reserves.

Follow the Asian Path

Indian political economy was on the wrong track for the first 40 years after independence. Asian countries that had also gone through the experience of colonialism had developed a small but vibrant nationalist business sector. They followed the Japanese model and harnessed their business leaders to the national growth agenda. Japan set the pattern for South Korea, Singapore, Taiwan and Hong Kong, who were hailed as the Asian Tigers in the 1970s. These were followed by Malaysia, Indonesia and even Vietnam. China abandoned its Leninist dogma after Mao's death and took off during the 1980s.

Among the colonial nations, India had the largest private industrial economy at the time of its independence, and was ranked as the seventh largest industrial nation. But the nationalist ideology wanted to believe that Britain had deindustrialized India and that only a state-led socialist policy was the way forward. So the nationalist private business sector was spurned, treated with suspicion, and accused of monopolistic and restrictive practices. Spurning the agro-based industrialization model advocated by Arthur Lewis as well as some Indian economists, such as C.N. Vakil and P.R. Brahmananda, the Soviet path of heavy machine-making was chosen, which generated few jobs. The open economy option was also rejected. Export pessimism and import substitution were the norms. Agriculture was taken for granted through the first two Five Year Plans. India stagnated with an average per capita growth rate of a mere 1 per cent for the first 30 years after independence.

An attempt to accelerate growth during the 1980s by borrowing from NRIs and import liberalization without reform of the Permit License Raj meant that while the economy boomed, it was a candyfloss growth. The crash of 1991, when India had to beg for a loan from IMF by pawning its gold reserves, was the supreme humiliation that arose from the faulty economics of all those years.

The decision to change course and re-enter the modern world in 1991 was much criticized. The then PM, P.V. Narasimha Rao, has never been nationally honoured nor his contribution acknowledged by his own party.

The BJP coming to power in 1998 ignored their protectionist lobby—the Swadeshi Jagaran Manch—and kept on the growth track as did the Congress upon returning to power in 2004. We have had growth till recently despite the cycle that began in 2016. The cure to that cycle is not unknown but requires firm policymaking and implementation. Even so, the protectionist noises are being heard louder during Modi 2.0. There are again demands for national self-sufficiency, small industries, etc., in a replay of the Congress text of the 1950s and 1960s. COVID has exposed the cost of slow growth, which leaves people underemployed or unemployed.

India is being given a second chance. It must have people-centred growth, not to make poverty tolerable as the old Gandhian economists wanted but with healthy lives and secure income-generating employment. Only a *suit-boot ki sarkar*[57] can clothe its people adequately.

It can be done. Look eastwards to the miracle economies of Asia, which started poorer than India in 1947 but have a per capita income several times higher than the India of today. They did so by exporting via their private sector and using government support strategically. India has to regain the momentum it had in 1991–2016. It will need another quarter century of high single-digit growth to enter the world of middle-income nations. What matters is not India's rank in terms of total GDP. A lot of people with low incomes and a few large fortunes have been India's story through the ages. India should have high per capita income and safe and secure livelihoods for its billion-and-a-half people by 2040. India needs to fix the long-run structural failures exposed by COVID if it is to grow, as it deserves to, and as many of its Asian neighbours—Japan, South Korea, Singapore, Indonesia, Malaysia—have successfully done.

◆

Meghnad Desai is emeritus professor of Economics at the London School of Economics, UK.

---

[57]Roughly translating to a corporate sector-friendly government.

TRADE POLICY

TRADE POLICY AND POST-COVID GROWTH

Jayanta Roy

COVID-19 struck India on top of an economic downturn, leading to the lowest national income growth in decades. I have argued in several places that this downturn was further accentuated as a result of the absence of structural reforms in a coordinated fashion. The present government abandoned trade reforms by the continuous imposition of tariffs, making the economy internationally non-competitive.

We made remarkable progress in trade and logistics facilitation, but did not follow it up with full speed. We have not yet succeeded in any mega-regional trade agreements, nor do we have a strong, deep and bilateral free trade agreement (FTA) with any major country. Our entire services sector is confined to IT and IT-enabled services and not diversified despite potentials of diversification. Our focus on FDI is not towards outward-oriented FDI, which is essential for technology transfer. Our institutional framework, with trade policy run by the antiquated Ministry of Commerce and Ministry of External Affairs, is not equipped to frame and implement trade policy, which now covers a long list of ministries and agencies related to all key aspects of trade policy.

Our big industries need to be confident to play the lead role in new neighbouring value chains that are in focus in the post-COVID world after major disruptions caused by it. This would help India to use its mature engineering sector integrated with lower-cost champions of intermediates in Vietnam, Thailand and other Southeast Asian countries, and manufacture the finished products in India. Pune, Chennai and Ahmedabad's innovative clusters would be able to integrate value chains across Southeast Asia, and deliver value-added final products to the global markets. Automation and trade tensions, and the near collapse of global value chains (GVCs) will certainly move the world fast towards neighbouring value chains, at least for a while. India needs to benefit from that by fully participating in it.

Before we discuss trade reforms needed to combat post-COVID disruptions, let us consider the reforms we need to carry out in trade policy to promote a rapid growth of sustained exports, which is necessary for creating jobs and achieving high and inclusive growth.

Trade Policy Recommendations for India that Are Long Overdue

The key to increasing Indian manufacturing exports is to integrate manufacturing into global production networks. The critical elements of policy required to integrate into the global supply chain are: a) relatively low tariffs (to allow easy importation of intermediates) and a simplified tariff structure, b) a regulatory environment that is attractive to FDI in manufacturing, c) a taxation system that ensures that no domestic taxes are exported (i.e., zero-rating of exports), d) an environment of low transaction costs of operating across borders, and e) strong logistical linkages, especially with regional economies. India currently lacks the comprehensive reform initiatives to achieve any of the five above-mentioned critical elements. A basic policy objective to integrate into regional production chains in Southeast Asia should be to bring Indian applied tariff levels down to the levels achieved by major ASEAN economies (from

14 percent to 9 percent, closer to the rate prevailing in ASEAN countries).

Integrating into international production chains also requires a domestic taxation system that is relatively transparent, stable, simple and ensures that no element of domestic tax is passed on to exports. It is obvious that if the added cost of domestic taxes is passed on to the price of the exported product, it will make such products less attractive for procurement within a price-sensitive global supply chain.

The introduction in July 2017 of a long-overdue comprehensive nationwide GST, the Indian version of Value-Added Tax, to replace a complicated domestic tax structure is an excellent move in this direction. A related demand has been the removal of all state and local taxes that are not rebated to exporters to ensure complete zero-rating of exports in terms of domestic taxes. Also, very soon the government should have a low, single uniform tax rate across the country to make it a common market.

Tariff policy alone will not be sufficient. Simultaneously, we need to urgently push the trade and logistics facilitation reforms, which are another big constraint to the rapid growth of exports and FDI, and the connectivity to GVCs. But to the credit of PM Modi, considerable reforms were undertaken during his tenure in this particular area, which are reflected in sharp improvements in the rankings of World Bank's Ease of Doing Business to 63, Trading across the Borders to 68 and Logistics Performance Indicators to 44. But, considerable improvements are still needed in these areas since India still lags behind most successful Southeast Asian countries (Table 1).

The PMEAC brought out a report in October 2018, outlining a clear road map for further reforms in trade and logistics facilitation. The key recommendations are:

TABLE 1
Doing Business and Logistics Facilitation indicators

Country	Doing Business Rank (2020)	Logistics Facilitation Rank (2019)
South Korea	5	25
Malaysia	12	41
Taiwan	15	27
Thailand	21	32
China	31	26
India	63	44
Vietnam	70	39
Bangladesh	168	100

Source: Doing Business and Logistics Performance Index Database-World Bank

Behind the Border Logistics

- Rationalizing rail tariff rationalization and expediting the commissioning of dedicated freight corridors
- Fast-tracking elimination of container freight stations and inland container depots by pushing direct port delivery (DPD) and direct port export (DPE)
- Nudging shipping lines to institute a transparent tariff structure
- Ensuring a seamless and efficient road transport experience—introduce a One Nation, One Permit, One Tax System
- Making business processes uniform and standardizing gate-in/gate-out approvals and documentation processes
- 24 × 7 shipping line services to trade
- Digitization and assessment of the automatic/digitization

At the Border Trade Facilitation

- Fully facilitated trust-based clearance processes through modern risk management systems
- Fully automated paperless trade environment with minimum face-to-face interactions
- Single-window digital portal integrating all stakeholders
- Monitoring of all key outputs across all major gateways
- Physical inspection of goods to be an exception
- Training of officers to operate/manage the new system, implement audit-based controls with the use of IT
- Popularize advance bills of entry, authorized economic operators, DPD and DPE in the private sector
- Target cargo dwell time to reach levels comparable to the successful Southeast Asian countries

Institutional Framework

- Establish a national council of logistics and trade facilitation outside the line ministries reporting to the PM
- To consist of cabinet ministers of the ministries and departments related to logistics and trade facilitation, and CMs of concerned states
- Private sector and trade stakeholders to be represented
- The Logistics wing presently under the Commerce Ministry be made a dedicated secretariat
- Development of robust performance outcomes for logistics and trade facilitation
- Monitor performance through an online dashboard and fix responsibilities for time-bound, corrective action
- Facilitate policy development and multi-stakeholder coordination
- Regular publication and dissemination of data on key sectoral outputs

Strong Potential of India Emerging as a Powerful GVC Hub

India should quickly implement these reforms to better connect to GVCs and revive the lost export momentum to spur high, inclusive growth and create jobs. India has the potential to benefit from GVCs, based on a number of advantages and opportunities, including the following:

- India has a very dynamic professional services sector and a very remarkable technology capacity, which are essential for task-oriented GVCs.
- India is yet a small player in GVCs with much room to grow. Its small and medium enterprises hardly participate in GVCs unlike those in Southeast Asia, China, South Korea, Japan, Mexico and some East European countries.
- The same is true for the levels of FDI, especially efficiency-seeking FDI, linked to creating a hub in India, which is at a dismally low level until now. Most of our FDI is market-seeking, catering to a large domestic market.
- India is ideally placed to be a supply chain hub, given its proximity to the high-growth Southeast Asia and East Asia.
- Most importantly, India has a government that has embarked on a sound foreign policy, which just needs to be complemented with matching deeper trade reforms outlined in this paper. The limited flow of outward-oriented FDI—which is needed for India to be a global and regional GVC hub—deserves attention. So does India's dismal performance in regional trade agreements.

FDI Linkage

Encouraging FDI Linkage with Production Networks

- Most FDI inflows into India have been a means of accessing the Indian consumer base
- FDI into an economy can have two motivations: Outward-looking FDI seeks to leverage competitiveness in certain aspects of a global supply chain to develop export-oriented manufacturing; and inward-looking FDI seeks to tap a large domestic market. If tariffs and costs of trading across borders of an economy are high, then FDI (i.e., investing in domestic production units) becomes the only vehicle through which a large domestic market can be accessed by foreign firms.
- Perception-based 'attractiveness' of India as an FDI destination is largely due to the size of the Indian market (inward-looking FDI). Scope of value-addition and network linkages are limited.
- While 100 per cent FDI is allowed in most sectors, the sheer number, complexity and scale of permits and approvals required from various levels of government, and poor logistics and business facilitation deters investors
- Reforms and single-window initiatives so far have promised much and delivered little
- Serious need to address issues related to time-bound decision-making and accountability of bureaucracy

Strategic Regionalism

- Energies are being dissipated in too many agreements that have little incremental value. These agreements also tend to be 'shallow' and do not address challenges of technical barriers and modern-day trade in a serious way.
- India should focus on Asia, especially greater southern Asia,

which includes South Asia and the ASEAN region. The Regional Comprehensive Economic Partnership (RCEP) and the Comprehensive and Progressive Agreement for Trans-Pacific Partnership (CPTPP) comprising the 11 original members of the Trans-Pacific Partnership (TPP), excluding the US (they are: Japan, Australia, New Zealand, Brunei, Singapore, Malaysia, Canada, Peru, Chile, Mexico and Vietnam) deserve attention.

- RCEP and CPTPP together address close to half of the global trade flows in goods. It is in this context that the government's decision to pull out of the RCEP agreement to be signed in 2020 is a cause of great concern. Hopefully, it is just a negotiating move, which will ultimately lead to India joining the RCEP. Indian industry will need to find ways to combat unfair Chinese trade practices as other member countries are doing.
- CPTPP, and to a much lesser extent, RCEP, represent trade agreements designed to address deeper twenty-first century trade issues and barriers. Although Donald Trump pulled US out of the TPP, which was initiated by his predecessor, it is quite possible that the US will eventually join CPTPP. India, in any case, should begin preparing to meet the WTO and trade policy requirements of CPTPP, to not only be a part of its vast value chain, but these policy reforms are also needed for India to emerge as a major global player. Once the US rejoins TPP, this then could emerge as the optimum trade deal between India and the US. Even to work out an effective FTA with the EU and the US, India needs to follow deep regionalism like the US has with Mexico and Canada (the US–Mexico–Canada Agreement [USMCA]), and like the EU has with Japan and Canada.
- Both these agreements will allow India to address important geo-economic goals and provide strategic depth; i.e., allow India to become a player of substance in the emerging Asian

architecture and the Indo-Pacific region.
- India also needs to start putting together a proactive trade policy strategy for Iran and seek deeper engagement with Africa, especially the Indian Ocean-African states.
- India also needs to turn its attention to seriously investing in and assisting Iran and Myanmar to create corridors of connectivity that work for India (to the rest of ASEAN via Myanmar, and central Asia and Eurasia via Iran).

Diversification of Professional Services

To benefit from GVCs, India has to diversify professional services beyond IT and IT-enabled services to other professional services. These are:

- Task-based value chain in professional services
  - Accounting, engineering, architecture, design, product development, legal and medical services are globally delivered, combining tasks being done by professionals in various locations
  - Each of the above has discrete tasks within the profession that can be outsourced; e.g., recording book entries, cleaning of accounts, analytics, tax-related assessment can all be unbundled to provide the final audit services. Trade policy to ensure maximum market access for all tasks within the profession and recognition of Indian qualifications.
- The analytics of big data, a huge emerging opportunity, will have its own skill-based value chain, with tasks ranging from basic quantitative assessment and presentation to the most advanced statistical and mathematical analysis.
- Tasks in social media and animation will move away from pure media and entertainment to multiple uses, ranging from training, education, real-time instruction modules

for decentralized manufacturing, and manuals for various products. This will create a range of professional services tasks.

In this context of strengthening GVC participation, we also need to focus on initiatives to facilitate India's place in the emerging value chain of digital and data-led service tasks. The policy interventions needed are as follows:

- Data protection and privacy issues can emerge as barriers. We need to engage our main trade partners through deeper trade agreements.
- Proactive reforms for the regulatory architecture of professional services, such as accounting, law, medical, architecture and engineering.
- Developing a regulatory architecture for newly developing professional services.
- In addition, there is a need to reduce transaction costs of service delivery from India by:
    - Reducing the cost of electricity, and ensuring 24×7 power supply
    - Reducing the cost of communication
    - Ensuring physical security
    - Availing certification for security and quality from foreign organizations (there are no national-level agencies in India)

We also need a new paradigm of education to create skill pipeline. My recommendations are:

- Transform three-year undergrad courses to create 2+2 options that focus on skills needed for the next generation of professional services
- Develop technical schools in public–private partnership mode, which allow students to develop job-specific

expertise for different tasks within the professional services value chain

Specific Trade Policy Focus in Post-COVID Recovery Period

As the COVID crisis rages on with no signs of abating, there is a need for some serious introspection on the toolkit of policies that will support India's post-COVID economic revival. While Atmanirbhar Bharat has provided some goalposts for a domestic industrial revival, there is lack of clarity on India's strategy for engaging the global economy. A sustained 8 per cent-plus economic growth cannot be achieved without having a successful and competitive export sector. Thus, an honest discussion on the challenges and options for Indian policymakers on trade is imperative.

But before delving into the details, it is important to first set the context, i.e., briefly describe the overall trade landscape in terms of products and markets, and the critical trade policy challenges India is likely to confront as the full spectrum of the COVID crisis and post-COVID economic realignment plays out.

Trade Landscape

- India's overall export of goods for April–June 2020 declined by about 37 per cent compared to the same period in the previous year. The decline for imports was at a much higher 52 per cent. These extremely sharp declines show the magnitude of supply chain disruptions and increasing impact of income shock from this crisis. The declines for services exports at about 10 per cent and import at about 19 per cent are lesser in magnitude but indicative of headwinds in near term.
- If one considers the overall structure of India's trade using data from the last three years or so, the country is a significant

player in the petroleum products and gems and jewellery value chains. It is both a large consumer and an exporter of value-added products. These two sectors account for a quarter of total exports and almost half of imports, and the COVID-induced income shock on these two sectors in the public–private partnership mode, which allow disproportionate effect on India's trade numbers. But the good news is that outside these sectors, India's export basket is quite diversified.

- India has also done well over the years in terms of market diversification. Using data from FY19, in the case of exports, apart from the US (17 per cent) and China plus Hong Kong (9 per cent), India is more or less evenly spread out in terms of market share. In imports, China plus Hong Kong accounts for a whopping 17 per cent of total imports, with US a distant second at 7 per cent, the remaining 74 per cent being more or less evenly spread out among other major trading partners. Given the geostrategic situation and the COVID-induced crisis, the elephants in the room are definitely China and the US.
- As highlighted before, India's services exports continue to remain overfocused on basic IT and IT-enabled services. This is under increasing strain as automation and robotics are rapidly eliminating many of the job roles in this segment. India needs to diversify into domain knowledge-based services, such as analytics, law, telemedicine, database management and security, artificial intelligence (AI) applications and many more. Labour-intensive work, such as data labelling, which enables unstructured data to be used for AI applications, in itself provides a huge opportunity.

Trade Challenges

- The COVID crisis has accelerated the process of the gradual erosion of Uruguay Round system of governance. While the

full extent of systemic damage is yet to be ascertained, it is clear that the WTO institutional mechanism is unlikely to provide the solutions to the rising tide of protectionism.
- WTO was designed to resolve trade disputes, not raging trade wars. It was also not designed to handle the legitimate grievances, with the trade-distorting measures and anti-competitive policies that have been used consistently by China at the detriment of other member states. As the expectation of China reforming its system and stopping predatory practices becomes increasingly less likely, and governments across the world face an economic crisis, patience is running out. The US–China trade war is only a symptom of this larger crisis.
- India has a lot to be concerned about. In many cases, the technical barriers to trade (TBTs) designed to counter China by major economies will also impact Indian exporters. Such TBTs in manufacturing and agriculture will increase the cost of compliance for Indian exporters, many of whom are small and medium enterprises. Unlike many competitor countries, such as like Thailand, Malaysia, Turkey or Mexico, India did not invest significantly in creating mechanisms that focus on reducing the cost of compliance for such technical standards for its exporters.
- The post-COVID world will not be conducive to the movement of people to deliver services (or Mode 4). Increasing digitalization due to COVID and reliance on e-delivery of work means electronic cross-border delivery of services (or Mode 1) would increase in importance. The Indian trade policy establishment obsession with Mode 4 needs to be given a long-overdue burial. To remain relevant in the services space, India needs to anticipate the new-age barriers in Mode 1. Such barriers include restrictions on the movement of data across borders, tariffication of digital delivery of services or other means to tax offshore data processing and other IT and

digital services. Behind the border restrictions of services related to professional standards, certifications, etc., remain firmly in place and can become more ubiquitous for a wider range of services.

Solutions

- India needs to get its act together. Solutions for TBTs and addressing emerging regulatory barriers in services cannot be done without a specific intent to engage major trading partners seriously. It also cannot be done within a low-ambition regional agreement, such as the RCEP. The geopolitical impact of China's conflicts with India, Japan and Australia will also take a toll on RCEP. This means India needs to refocus itself on the ambitious CPTPP, and bilateral agreements with deep regionalism focus with the US and the UK. Looking at the USMCA and EU FTAs with Japan and South Korea, the task will pose great challenges to Indian industry, which is not yet geared up for international competition as a result of governments maintaining protectionist policies.
- There is an urgent need to start exploring trade deals with the US and the EU, and find ways to address the TBTs and services market access more comprehensively in existing agreements with Japan, South Korea and ASEAN member states. But this cannot be done if India's atmanirbharta[58] translates into protectionism. India would need to confidently offer market access in areas of interest to trade partners as it seeks concessions for its own industrial interests.
- Negotiating with more advanced economies is much easier since there is likely to be a large number of areas where their advanced industrial sectors are either churning out products that do not have local competitors or represent a higher-

---

[58]Self-sufficiency

price-higher-quality option. Doing this successfully requires a thorough understanding of India's sector-by-sector strengths and weaknesses and a genuine industrial development policy that strategically identifies long-term value-chain ambitions for key sectors in India. Such analytical homework is sorely missing today. This lacuna is the result of not investing in a robust trade policy cell staffed with professional trade economists and trade specialists in the Ministry of Commerce and Industry. This needs to be rectified urgently.

- Ad hoc attempts and occasional jamborees, such as the India–Africa or the Bay of Bengal Initiative for Multi-Sectoral Technical and Economic Cooperation (BIMSTEC) summits, need to be replaced with credible South Asian and African trade and investment plans. Such plans would have a list of actionable items that combine trade policy incentives, outward FDI strategies for Indian firms to leverage these growing markets, and dovetailing development aid and technical assistance programmes to help Indian exports. This actionable agenda would have deadlines and would be accountable to a special officer in the PM's Office (PMO), who will follow through with the different ministries and industry associations on the progress of the plan and submit regular reports to the PMO for review. The actionable agenda could include entering into FTAs with African and BIMSTEC countries.
- India would also need a strategy for the structural overhaul of its services export sector. Its large domestic market for digital services and very large absolute numbers of a college-educated workforce gives it an edge. It needs to use its diaspora networks in the global technology sector and start-up ecosystem to ramp itself up in the GVC to develop India-based service solutions around Internet of Things (IoT), AI and AI-based applications, and data analytics.

- Last but not the least, India needs to get really ambitious on Trade Facilitation. Jumping from a rank of below 100 to 67 in the World Bank's Doing Business across borders shows that the Modi government has the right intentions. But there is still regulatory overhang in a number of areas that allows too much ad hoc decision-making by customs officials, relatively poor use of risk management, leading to high percentages of shipments being heaped up for processing at gateway ports, and delayed rebate of duties and taxes that negatively impact cash flows of exporting businesses.

This paper lays out clearly the specific trade policy reforms the government needs to initiate and implement, starting as soon as possible. Their success is predicated upon a trade institutional framework that places a small national trade policy council that reports to the PM, and which is outside the line ministries. We urgently need an institutional reform for trade policy. We need our PM to be directly involved with the new institutions. Our PM has shown his leadership by single-handedly overcoming our poor business climate and massive trade transaction costs. We now need him to oversee trade negotiations, continue with trade and logistics reforms, and make our economy competitive.

Given the cross-cutting nature of the twenty-first century trade agenda, leadership should not rest with any line ministry. What is needed is an 'apex entity' that has a clear mandate from the PM to consult with stakeholders and manage the process of developing the strategy. This entity cannot be solely responsible for implementation as that will by necessity involve many players in and outside the government. Instead, its role in the implementation phase is to act as coordinator and convener, and to have the mandate to monitor and assess implementation by relevant agencies within the government.

The proposed national trade policy council will ensure that all agencies that are involved with trade activities—line ministries, regulatory bodies, state governments—know what the goals are. They are fully informed of the priorities that are defined by the strategy, and use it as a framework that guides their activities.

The national trade policy council should be chaired by a minister who reports directly to the PM. It should include senior representatives of all relevant ministries and regulatory agencies. It should have the mandate to create technical committees that bring together sectoral or issue-specific experts to provide inputs on the design or implementation of specific dimensions of the trade strategy. It could have two offices—office of the chief trade negotiator, and the national council of logistics and trade facilitation. Trade policy needs to be on the radar screen of the PM.

♦

Jayanta Roy was economic advisor, Ministry of Commerce, Government of India in 1991 when India initiated trade liberalization. He has been the regional lead economist at the World Bank, and principal adviser on Trade and Globalization to the Confederation of Indian Industry. He has taught at the World Bank Institute; Cornell University; the University of California, Santa Cruz; the University of Warwick, UK; and the Indian Institute of Management, Calcutta.

EXPLAINING INDIA'S TRADE PERFORMANCE

Biswajit Dhar

Six months since the government announced the lockdown in an effort to prevent the spread of COVID-19, the Indian economy seems to be settling into a long road to recovery, putting behind its worst-ever quarterly performance in the first quarter of 2020–21. Unfortunately for India, the pandemic made its impact felt when its economy was on a downward spiral for eight consecutive quarters, during which the growth of GDP had declined from 7.1 per cent in the first quarter of financial year 2018–19 to 3.1 per cent in the fourth quarter of 2019–20. This outcome resulted from the fact that the two critical growth drivers, namely, investment and exports, had registered negative growth rates in all the quarters of 2019–20, except in the first quarter, while consumption demand had barely expanded. These three growth drivers were at their historical lows in Q1 2020–21, pushing GDP to contract by almost 24 per cent over the corresponding period in 2019–20.

Exports have been one of the low points of India's economic performance, especially during the previous decade. Over the past three decades, the economy was opened up with the expectation that exposing domestic producers to international competition would improve their efficiencies, enabling them to increase their presence in the global markets. This process was given further momentum through the implementation of three

FTAs, with several high-performing economies in East Asia during the previous decade. But despite following the policies of openness, the country's exports remained largely subdued, while imports expanded as the partner countries took advantage of an increasingly open Indian economy. The country that made its presence felt the most was China, which emerged as India's import source.

This chapter discusses India's trade performance since the turn of the millennium and dwells on some of the key features, the most prominent of these being the growing role of China. I would explain the pattern of India–China trade, alluding to the main areas of India's dependence on its northern neighbour.

The second section of the paper provides some explanations of the pattern of India's trade in general and with China in particular. This section would discuss the possible policy options to address the problems that have plagued India's export performance.

India's Trade Performance in the New Millennium

India entered the new millennium as one of the lesser-integrated economies with the global economy on a number of counts. First, India's average tariffs on a most favoured nation basis was nearly 34 per cent in the year 2000, which was relatively high as compared to most advanced developing economies. Secondly, India's trade-to-GDP ratio in 1999–2000 was over 26 per cent, up from just above 20 per cent in 1992–93, when the process of economic liberalization was initiated. And finally, India's share in global trade was nearly stagnant in the 1990s, increasing to 0.7 per cent in the year 2000 from 0.6 per cent in 1991.

In the new millennium, the situation changed considerably in terms of trade openness, as Table 1 shows. Tariffs on industrial products were lowered sharply, from an average of 31 per cent in 2000 to below 9 per cent just when the Great Recession of 2008 had struck. Tariffs on agricultural products were also reduced but were well above those for industrial products. Since then, import duties have remained at this level, until they were increased in 2018.[59]

TABLE 1
Simple average tariffs on agricultural and industrial products (in %)

Years	Agricultural Products*	Industrial Products*
1992**	48.9	57.5
2000	40.1	30.5
2003	36.9	24.8
2005	37.6	15.4
2008	32.2	8.9
2009	38.8	10.1
2010	31.4	9.0
2015	32.8	9.8
2017	32.7	9.9
2018	38.8	13.3
2019	38.8	14.1

Notes: *based on WTO's classification of products; ** figures from Trade Analysis Information System database

Sources (for Tables 1 & 2): WTO Integrated Database, obtained from the World Integrated Trade Solution

---

[59] India's average import duties for industrial products were between 9 and 11 per cent until 2018. A series of duty increases in 2018 raised the average import duties to 14 per cent.

Biswajit Dhar. (2019). 'India's Withdrawal from the Regional Comprehensive Economic Partnership', Economic & Political Weekly November 16, Vol LIV No 45; pp. 59-65.

Coinciding with tariff reduction, India's merchandise trade began to show greater dynamism from the beginning of the millennium (Chart 1). However, figures for the two decades presented in the figure show sharply contrasting trade performance. In the first phase, exports grew by an annual average of over 17 per cent and imports expanded by over 22 per cent. This helped in increasing India share in global trade from 0.7 per cent in the year 2000 to 1.5 per cent in 2010. But in the second phase, growth of both exports and imports shrank to below 7 per cent, and India's share in global trade was pegged at 2.1 per cent in 2019.

Chart 1: India's trade performance (2000–01 to 2018–19)

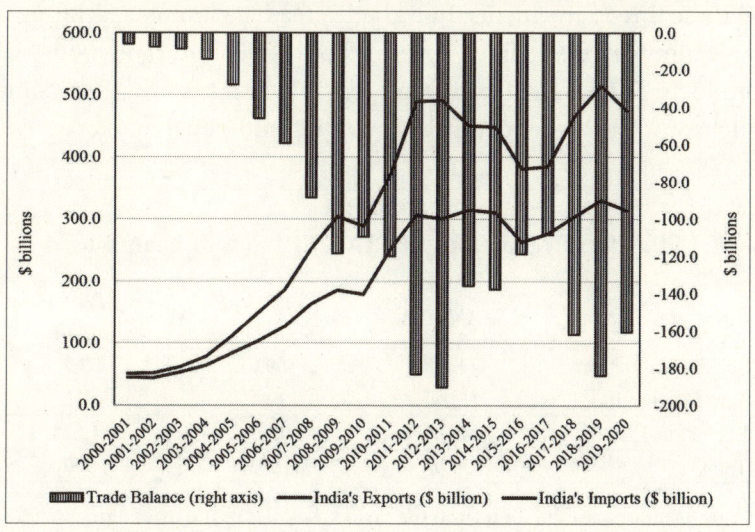

Source: Directorate General of Commercial Intelligence and Statistics, Department of Commerce.

The above trends show two interesting facets: first, the period of tariff liberalization in the 2000s was accompanied by rising levels of trade, though imports expanded faster than exports, and secondly, trade flows remained pegged to a narrow range in the previous decade when import tariffs remained unchanged, except for the two most recent years. There is, however, an important counter-factual that must also be considered while examining the relationship between lowering of tariffs liberalization and trade flows. This pertains to India's experience with the implementation of comprehensive economic partnership agreements (CEPAs), which were formalized with three partners, namely the ASEAN members, South Korea and Japan, which we shall briefly discuss below.

Implementation of CEPAs and the Trends of Trade Flows

In these three agreements, India had agreed to eliminate tariffs on a large number of tariff lines, covering both agricultural and industrial products (Table 2). It was expected that exports would become buoyant with partner countries providing additional market access.

TABLE 2
India's tariff reductions in FTA/CEPAs (% of tariff lines)

Categories	ASEAN FTA	CEPA with South Korea	CEPA with Japan
Tariff Elimination	74.2	69.7	87.7
Tariff Reduction	15.1	14.1	NIL
Exclusion List	10.7	16.2	12.3
Total	100.0	100.0	100

Source: Author's compilation from the tariff schedules of the three agreements

The three agreements were adopted between 2009 and 2011 and have almost been implemented.[60]

Chart 2 shows India's trade patterns with the CEPA partners.

---

[60]Cambodia, Lao People's Democratic Republic (Laos), Myanmar and Vietnam will fully implement their commitments to an open market for Indian goods by 2021.

Chart 2: Trade with FTA/CEPA partners

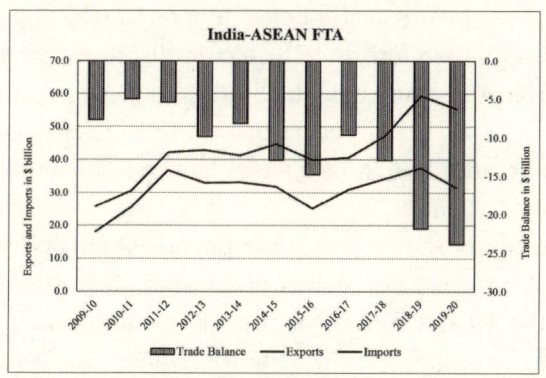

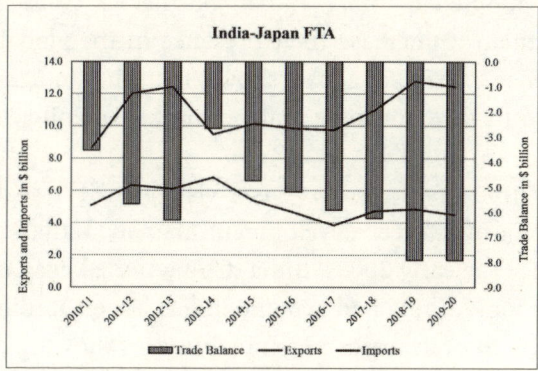

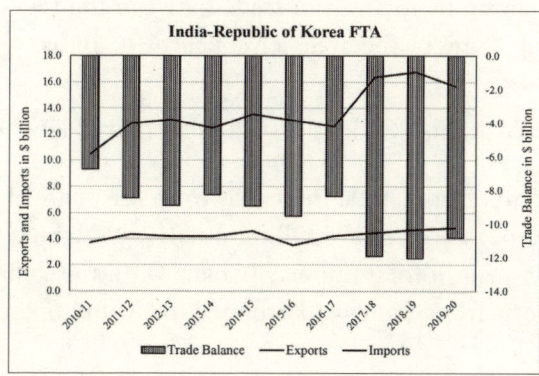

Source: Directorate General of Commercial Intelligence and Statistics, Department of Commerce.

The implementation of these agreements has shown that India's partners were able to secure better market access opportunities, and they were, therefore, able to secure disproportionately large benefits from these agreements. Studies have shown that India's trade deficit vis-à-vis all three partners have increased consistently, especially because Indian businesses have not been able increase their exports[61] (Chart 2).

Our analysis shows that trade liberalization policy, initially a unilateral process, which was given fillip since the mid-2000s through the FTAs/CEPAs, was unable to sufficiently stimulate exports. As mentioned earlier, the trade liberalization agenda in 1991 was adopted to make Indian businesses competitive and to enable them to increase their presence in the global markets. The evidence provided above shows that the Indian industry was unable to take advantage of the market opening in partner countries.

India's trade performance vis-à-vis the CEPA partners was but a subplot of a larger development, namely, India's trade with China. Since the early 2000s, India–China trade began expanding and before long, China had become India's largest trading partner on the strength of its exports to India. In the following discussion we will examine the pattern of trade between the two countries, highlighting some of the areas of concern for India.

Patterns of India–China Trade Since the Early 2000s

India's imports from China increased from less than $3 billion in 2002–03 to peak at over $76 billion in 2017–18, which was more than 16 per cent of total imports (Chart 3). In the following two years, imports from China had dropped to $65 billion in 2019–20,

---

[61]Biswajit Dhar. (2018). 'India's Comprehensive Economic Partnership Agreements with ASEAN, Japan and Korea', Penang: Third World Network.

or nearly 14 per cent of total imports.

From an Indian perspective, the larger cause for concern was the inability of the exports to penetrate the Chinese market. India's exports peaked at $18 billion in 2012–13, but subsequently, they were pegged back to $13 billion in 2017–19, resulting in an increase in trade deficit to a massive $63 billion, or nearly 40 per cent of India's overall trade deficit. In the past two years, the trend of rising trade deficit reversed as India's exports expanded to $16 billion, while imports from China declined.

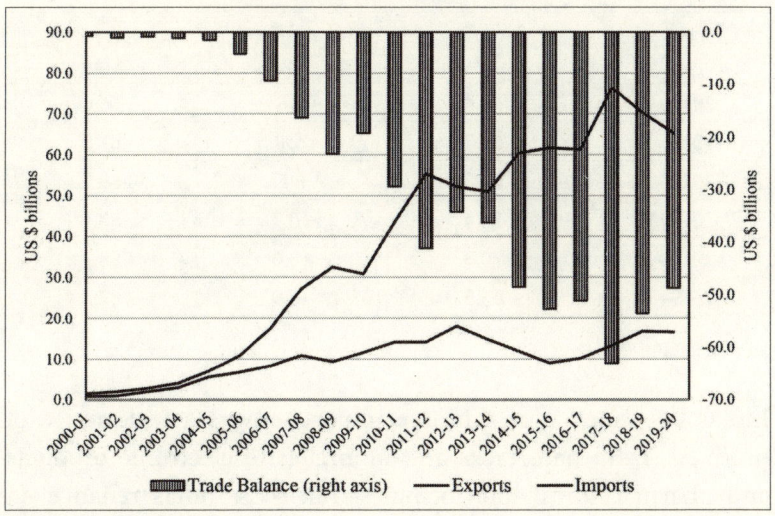

Chart 3: India–China trade

Source: Directorate General of Commercial Intelligence and Statistics, Department of Commerce.

Though imports from China reduced over the past two years, this may not be the reality as imports from Hong Kong increased in the meanwhile. Hong Kong has long served as the gateway for the distribution of China's products to the rest of the world. An earlier study reported that during 1988–98, 53 per cent of China's exports were distributed via Hong Kong.[62] In more recent years, some reports have indicated that there are other motivations, including tax avoidance, to rout Chinese exports through Hong Kong.[63] Increase in India's imports from Hong Kong needs to be seen in light of the aforementioned. In fact, the table below shows that the increase in imports from Hong Kong was more than compensating the decline in the imports from China; in effect, there was no real reduction in imports from China.

TABLE 3
India's imports from China and Hong Kong SAR ($ bn)

Years	China	Hong Kong	China + Hong Kong
2014–15	60.4	5.6	66.0
2015–16	61.7	6.1	67.8
2016–17	61.3	8.2	69.5
2017–18	76.4	10.7	87.1
2018–19	70.3	18.0	88.3
2019–20	65.3	16.9	82.2

Source: DGCI&S

India's dependence on Chinese imports covers a wide range of products, from nails/tacks and umbrellas to electronic products and pharmaceutical intermediates. But it is India's reliance on Chinese imports in two product groups, namely, telecom and

---

[62] Gordon H. Hanson, and Robert C. Feenstra. (2001). 'Intermediaries in Entrepot Trade: Hong Kong Re-Exports of Chinese Goods', NBER Working Paper No. 8088, accessed from: https://www.nber.org/papers/w8088.

[63] Jake Van Der Kamp. (2016). 'Taxing question of why China exports goods via Hong Kong', South China Morning Post, April 8, accessed from: https://www.scmp.com/comment/insight-opinion/article/1934945/taxing-question-why-china-exports-goods-hong-kong.

electronics products, and active pharmaceutical ingredients (APIs), which are particularly disconcerting given the criticality of these sectors for the Indian economy. The importance of telecom and electronics products have increased manyfold over the past few years after the government initiated the Digital India programme in 2015, which 'is a flagship programme of the Government of India with a vision to transform India into a digitally empowered society and knowledge economy'.[64] More important is India's dependence on China for APIs, which has helped the Indian generic manufacturers to provide cheap medicines, not only in India but to many countries in both developing and the developed world. Due to its deep penetration in the global markets, the Indian industry has acquired the sobriquet of the 'pharmacy of the world'.

Imports of electronic and telecommunications equipment from China have been quite significant. There is a common perception that fairly large volumes of mobile phones are sourced from China, which is indeed the case as more than 83 per cent of the imports were of Chinese origin in 2019–20. But the fact that during the same year, nearly 90 per cent of colour TV sets imported into the country were from this country should surprise most. More importantly, India continues to depend substantially on Chinese telecom transmission equipment.

The syndrome of dependence on China is considerably worse in case of APIs. In recent years, India has been depending exclusively on China for imports of paracetamol, the common antipyretic and anti-inflammatory medicine. Similarly, India was completely dependent on China for the imports of streptomycin and had high levels of dependence on other antibiotics, such as ciprofloxacin and amoxycillin. China has also been supplying the

---

[64]Government of India. (2015). Digital India Programme, accessed from: https://www.digitalindia.gov.in/

APIs for rifampicin, used for treating several bacterial infections, including tuberculosis.

From this syndrome of India's import dependence on China, two conclusions can be drawn. First, dependence of India's pharmaceutical industry on China shows that this industry has fairly weak foundations, which can be problematic for two reasons. While disruptions in supplies from China can seriously affect production, there is no assurance that the Chinese suppliers of APIs have been maintaining the quality of their products in conformity with the global standards. Secondly, since India imports more than 90 per cent of the APIs from China for several critical antibiotics and vitamins, it seems improbable that India can succeed in finding an alternate source for meeting its API requirements.

The list of other industries depending on China for their essential supplies is fairly long, but three sectors need mentioning. The first is the motorcycle industry, which, in 2018–19, sourced 85 per cent of its imports of the parts and components from China. While most of the motorcycle components are obtained locally, the industry imports critical parts, such as wheel rims, from China. Yet another disconcerting trend is that India is heavily dependent on China for solar photovoltaic cells; in 2019–20, more than 90 per cent of imports of silicon wafers and solar lanterns were of Chinese origin. The third sector is textiles, in which synthetic and artificial woven yarn imports from China have risen.

The commodity composition of India–China trade sums up the trade relations between the two countries as they have evolved over the past two decades. Charts 4 and 5 summarize the patterns of India's imports from and its exports to China as distributed between four broad product categories.

India's imports from China have increasingly been skewed towards capital goods, which include consumer durables, while imports of intermediates, such as APIs, have also been sizeable.

**Chart 4: Composition of India's imports from China
(% of total imports)**

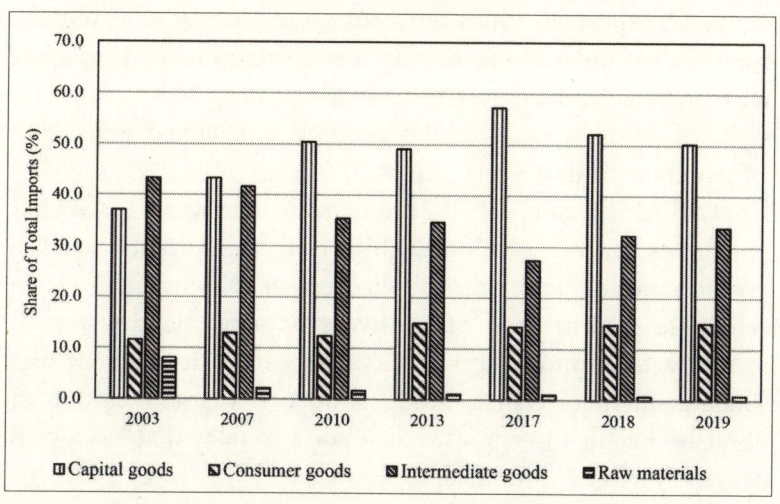

**Chart 5: Composition of India's exports to China
(% of total exports)**

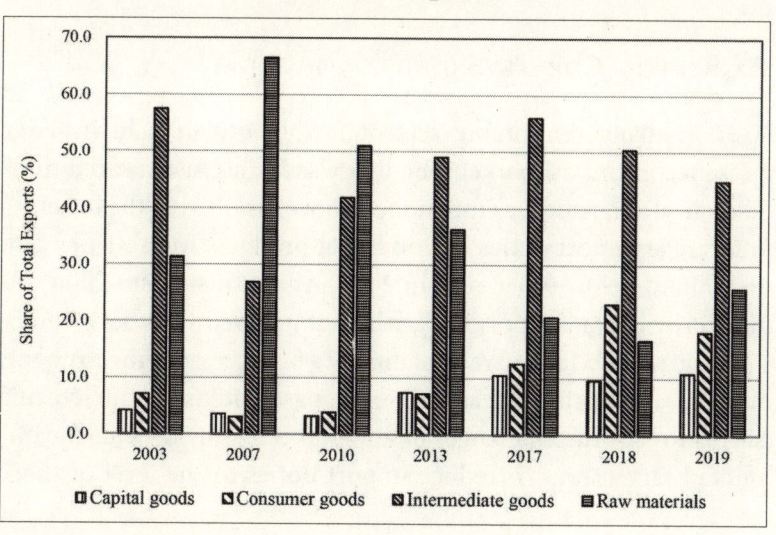

Sources for Chart 4 and 5: UN Comtrade Database

The share of these products increased from 37 per cent in 2003 to 57 per cent in 2017, after which it fell to 50 per cent in 2019 (Chart 4). India's exports to China are a complete contrast to its imports from China. India has largely been supplying raw materials and intermediate products to China since the early 2000s, while the share of consumer and capital goods has remained well below 30 per cent in most years (Chart 5).

Two conclusions can be drawn from the above discussion. The first is that vis-à-vis India, China is in a significantly superior position in the international division of labour. The relative economic performances of the two economies stand testimony to this fact. Secondly, from India's perspective, dependence on a single country for critical products in such a large measure can never be a right strategy, especially for a country that has a huge demand for these products.

What explains this sustained expansion of imports from China since the early 2000s and can India alter this trend? We shall briefly dwell on these issues below.

Explaining China's Expansion in India

Two mutually reinforcing sets of factors explain China's large presence in India's market. The first was India's fast-tracked trade liberalization, which, as mentioned above, resulted in the lowering of average import duties on industrial products from 31 per cent in 2000 to below 9 per cent in 2008. An expansionist China was thus provided an opportunity, which it grabbed with both hands.

The second factor was the inability of successive governments to take appropriate measures to prepare India's manufacturing sector to face the challenges of an open economy. One of the oft-quoted targets was to reduce import duties to the level of those adopted by the East Asian countries.⁶⁵ What was not given due importance was that these economies had adopted well-honed industrial policies, which had enabled their industries to not only face import competition in their increasingly open economies, but to also become globally competitive.

It was not as if advice on the urgent need to shore up the industrial sector was not forthcoming. In 2006, the National Manufacturing Competitiveness Council⁶⁶ advised the government to take prompt measures to raise the share of manufacturing in the country's GDP to 20 per cent within a decade. The UPA government unveiled the National Manufacturing Policy in 2011 in which the target set was to increase the share of manufacturing in GDP to 25 per cent within a decade.⁶⁷ And, finally, the Make in India initiative was launched in 2014 to strengthen the manufacturing sector and 'raising the contribution of the manufacturing sector' to 25 per cent of the GDP 'in the coming years'. But the share of manufacturing in GDP has remained stuck between 15 and 17 per cent for two reasons. One, the policy pronouncements for improving the share of the manufacturing sector in GDP were not backed up by concrete instruments, and two, in some of the key sectors, including electronics and pharmaceuticals, inappropriate instruments were adopted.

Production of electronic products in India goes back to the 1960s when public sector enterprises were tasked with the

---

⁶⁵Biswajit Dhar. (2020). 'Political Economy of India's Trade Liberalisation', in Johannes Plagemann, Sandra Destradi and Amrita Narlikar (eds.), India Rising: A Multilayered Analysis of Ideas, Interests, and Institutions. 176-207. New Delhi: Oxford University Press.
⁶⁶Government of India. (2006). The National Strategy for Manufacturing, National Manufacturing Competitiveness Council, New Delhi.
⁶⁷Government of India. (2011). National Manufacturing Policy, Press Note 2 (2011 Series), Ministry of Commerce and Industry, accessed from: https://dipp. gov.in/sites/default/files/po-ann4.pdf.

responsibility of producing computing devices.⁶⁸ Consumer electronics took roots in the following decade and a fledgling industry was in place by the time the policies of economic liberalization were introduced in 1991.⁶⁹

In the early phase of import liberalization, the electronics sector was largely kept out of this exercise, but the situation changed drastically after India, in 1996, joined the Information Technology Agreement (ITA), a plurilateral agreement under the WTO. When the ITA became effective on 1 July 1997, only 28 members⁷⁰ of the WTO had acceded to the agreement. According to the terms of the agreement, India agreed to eliminate import duties on 217 IT products by 2005. Consequently, India's average import duties on IT products came down from 66.4 per cent in the pre-ITA phase to 37.8 per cent in 1997 to below 12 per cent in 2001, before the tariffs were completely eliminated on 1 January 2005.

The rationale for India's accession to ITA seems difficult to understand as India was a minor player in the global market for ITA products. India's exports of IT products were the lowest among the 28 original signatories to the ITA between 1997 and 2003.⁷¹ In sharp contrast, China had become the third largest exporter of IT products in 2003, and Hong Kong was not far behind. In fact, China and Hong Kong taken together were the largest exporters of IT products from 2003 onwards. It was hardly surprising that rapidly developing Chinese enterprises would take

---

⁶⁸Biswajit Dhar. (2019). 'India's Withdrawal from the Regional Comprehensive Economic Partnership', Economic & Political Weekly November 16, Vol LIV No 45; pp. 59-65.
⁶⁹Subhrajit Guhathakurta. (1994). Electronics Policy and the Television Manufacturing Industry: Lessons from India's Liberalization Efforts. Economic Development and Cultural Change. Vol. 42, No. 4. pp. 845-868
⁷⁰EU members are counted as a single customs territory
⁷¹Based on author's estimates using UN Comtrade.

advantage of an open Indian market bereft of strong domestic competitors.

The case of dependence on China for APIs stems from the failure to ensure that domestic suppliers were available for an expanding formulations industry. This was not the outcome that policymakers in the immediate post-independence phase has envisioned. In 1954, the government had established the Hindustan Antibiotics Limited for producing penicillin and other antibiotics and vitamins.[72] The Indian Drugs and Pharmaceuticals Limited was established in 1961 to manufacture antibiotics, synthetic drugs and surgical instruments.[73]

In 1974, the Committee on Drugs and Pharmaceutical Industry (the 'Hathi Committee') was constituted to recommend, among others, measures 'necessary for ensuring that the public sector attains a leadership role in the manufacture of basic drugs (APIs) and formulations, and in research and development'.[74] The Hathi Committee recommended that a strong public sector along with the private sector would be essential for a resilient pharmaceutical industry in India. In subsequent decades, while the formulations sector expanded rapidly, every government, without exception, neglected the public sector enterprises that could have met the growing APIs' requirement. This demand–supply gap in APIs was fully exploited by the Chinese enterprises.

---

[72]Committee on Public Undertakings. (1976). Eightieth Report on Hindustan Antibiotics Limited. Fifth Lok Sabha. New Delhi: Lok Sabha Secretariat.
[73]Committee on Public Undertakings. (1969). Forty-Sixth Report: Indian Drugs and Pharmaceuticals Limited. Fourth Lok Sabha. New Delhi: Lok Sabha Secretariat.
[74]Ministry of Petroleum and Chemicals. (1975). The Committee on Drugs and Pharmaceutical Industry (Hathi Committee Report). Government of India.

Conclusion

India's trade performance over the past two decades has shown serious signs of weaknesses, stemming from the inability of the country's manufacturing sector to become globally competitive. In our discussion above, I have alluded to two major problems that a non-competitive manufacturing sector has given rise to. First, the manufacturing sector, which has contributed more than 87 per cent of India's total merchandise exports in recent years, has been unable increase its exports in any significant manner. Further, with domestic manufacturing unable to compete with imports in an increasingly open economy, unacceptably high levels of import dependence have developed in several critical sectors.

Although successive governments have announced policies for strengthening the manufacturing sector from the middle of the 2000s, appropriate policy instruments to back these announcements have largely been missing. In the post-COVID phase, one of the most important tasks for the government is to develop a medium-term strategy for the revival of the manufacturing sector. Such a strategy would be critically dependent on a coherent industrial policy, which must have the enabling conditions as well as the optimum level of incentives for the entrepreneurs. There is no gainsaying that trade can become an effective growth driver for the economy only when it is backed by competitive domestic producers.

◆

Biswajit Dhar is professor, Centre for Economic Studies and Planning at Jawaharlal Nehru University, New Delhi. He was formerly director general, Research and Information System for Developing Countries, and of the Centre for WTO Studies, Government of India. He has been a member of the Indian delegation at the World Trade Organization.

EMPLOYMENT AND MIGRATION

REVIVING MANUFACTURING AND EMPLOYMENT

R. Nagaraj

In 2019–20, the National Accounts Statistics 2020 shows, the Indian economy grew at 4.2 per cent, adjusted for inflation. The growth rate got nearly halved in less than three years since 2016–17. Concurrently, the manufacturing growth rate collapsed to zero from 6.6 per cent. If the doubts raised about the reliability of the official GDP have merit, the actual growth rate may be lower by 1–2 percentage points.[75]

By the turn of 2020, a clear picture of the economy in distress emerged, by piecing together the credible aggregate statistics.[76] The economy slowed down significantly after the boom years of 2003–08—the Dream Run, as I called it—that went bust by the early years of the 2010s. The disputed GDP estimates, however, have muddied the statistical picture for the last decade.

The growth slowdown has accompanied (i) an unprecedented decline in the aggregate fixed investment and saving rates as proportions of GDP, and (ii) a steady deceleration in bank credit growth, new investment approvals and industrial capacity utilization. Between 2011–12 and 2017–18, as per the National

---

[75]See Pramit Bhattacharya and Nikita Kwatra (2020). 'Getting the GDP Measurement Right', Livemint, July 27 for an up-to-date summary of the GDP estimation debate.
[76]R. Nagaraj. (2020). 'Understanding India's Economic Slowdown: Need for Concerted Action', The India Forum, February 7.

Sample Survey's estimates, (a) employment rate fell, and the open UR% rose to unprecedented levels (in urban areas in particular), (b) real wages declined, and (c) per capita personal consumption fell in real terms (mainly in rural India). Expectedly, therefore, the absolute poverty rate increased for the first time in nearly four decades.

There is a silver lining, though. The inflation rate, however measured, declined in the latter half of the 2010s. BoP deficit has also remained modest due to the collapse of global oil prices as the Great Recession has continued to bite. India is, thus, suffering from inadequate aggregate demand in the short to medium term, owing to a fall in the investments and exports as a proportion of GDP.

The Pandemic, Lockdown and Exposed Inherent Vulnerabilities

What has changed during the months since after the COVID-19 pandemic and the economic lockdown? Uncertainties about the nation's health and economic conditions have bogged down everyone, especially the poor and unemployed.

The lockdown imposed in end-March, with just four hours' notice, considered the world's most severe, was indeed an economic shock. The government hoped to catch the virus by its neck to minimize its spread. But the sudden lockdown sharply dislocated production and transportation, retrenched output and employment, most acutely in the non-farm informal sector. With the collapse of jobs and incomes, workers lost their rented living spaces in cities. With public transport shut down, migrant workers scrambled to get back to their villages, leading to a humanitarian crisis.

Even after nearly six months, without work and shelter, the urban poor continue to suffer. Social activist Harsh Mandar's field reports testify to how so many displaced workers are stuck in the fringes of Delhi living under flyovers in inhumane conditions.[77] Emergency efforts are on to meet the health pandemic, with little signs of the 'flattening of the curve', nationally. With the virus spreading to industrial towns and villages, economic revival after 'unlocking' since June is restricted by the spread of the virus (for instance, textile weaving centres of Bhiwandi or Solapur). Many states and cities have reimposed localized lockdowns in response, thus muting the economic recovery.

By early September, India had the world's second largest number of COVID-19 positive cases, though the recovery rate now exceeds two-thirds of the cases, and mortality rates are declining. However, health professionals seem sceptical about the integrity of the official estimates. Testing for the virus is inadequate in smaller cities and rural areas. Mortality numbers are reportedly from hospitals, not from crematoria and burial grounds by municipal authorities. As there is no chance for the virus disappearing overnight, we are indeed in it for the long haul. There are no quick fixes in sight, warranting more durable solutions. The pandemic has exposed India's long-term neglect of public health. Total government expenditure on health as a proportion of GDP is just about 1.3 per cent. A recent report by Oxfam said[78]:

> Towards the bottom of the overall health spending ranking is India, which has also made cuts to its health budget (albeit small) and has fallen to third-last position of this ranking. This is particularly damaging when just half of India's population has access to even the most essential services, and more than

---

[77] *The Hindu*, August 7, 2020
[78] Development Finance International and Oxfam. (2020). Fighting Inequality in the time of COVID-19: The Commitment to Reducing Inequality Index, October 2020

70% of health spending is being met from household budgets. This has left the country woefully ill-prepared to deal with the coronavirus pandemic.

The health pandemic also revealed India's limited manufacturing capacities of critical items and significantly rising dependence on Chinese imports for bulk drugs. The PM's call for Atmanirbhar Bharat during the lockdown, reiterated in the Independence Day address, seems a tacit admission of the growing external economic threat.

Economic Effects of the Pandemic

IMF WEO's June update says that global output has been forecasted to decline by 4.9 per cent in 2020–21, compared to the previous year—the worst since the Great Depression.[79] Likewise, WTO's press release in April 2020 said that it anticipates world merchandise trade to fall between 13 and 32 per cent in 2020, affecting all regions, commodities and sectors.[80]

India's quarterly GDP estimates for April–June 2020, released on August 31, show a contraction of 24 per cent over the same quarter last year. It is worst among the G20 countries on a comparable basis, as per IMF Chief Economist Gita Gopinath's tweeted data (Chart 1). The forecast for the full year 2020–21 is a decline in output level (or, a negative growth rate compared to the previous year) by 10.3 per cent, as per IMF WEO's October 2020 edition.

---

[79] IMF (2020): World Economic Outlook Update, June, (https://www.imf.org/en/Publications/WEO/Issues/2020/06/24/WEOUpdateJune2020), accessed on November 6, 2020.
[80] Trade set to plunge as COVID-19 pandemic upends global economy. (8 April 2020) Accessed from: https://www.wto.org/english/news_e/pres20_e/pr855_e.htm, on November 6, 2020.

Chart 1: GDP Growth

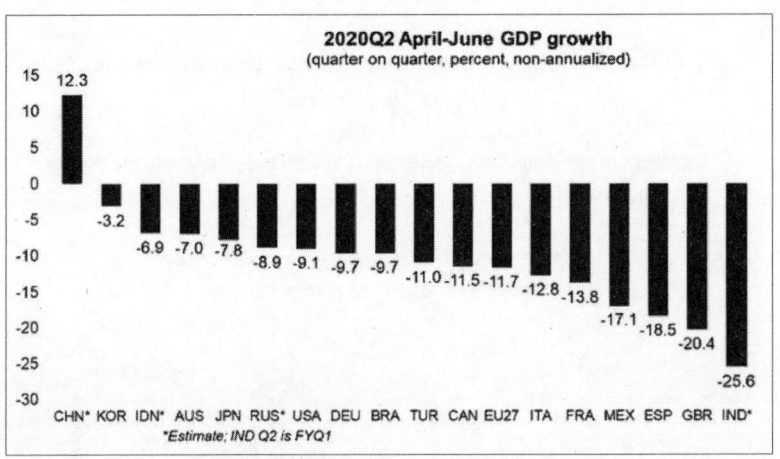

Source: IMF Chief Economist's tweet dated 2 September 2020

To mitigate the economic crisis, in May, the government announced its most substantial relief and revival package, known as Atmanirbhar Bharat, amounting to ₹20 lakh crore, or about 10 per cent of GDP. However, the package mostly consisted of liquidity support and credit guarantees (mostly conditional upon meeting reform criteria). Additional budgetary expenditure—as widely acknowledged—that would add to current aggregate spending is just about 1 percentage point of GDP.

Chart 2, from the IMF report mentioned above, shows that the 'additional spending and foregone revenue' in India is one of the lowest among the world's major countries, and even among emerging market economies.[81] India's efforts are smaller than Vietnam's at 3.5 per cent of GDP, as per a report of Oxford

---

[81] IMF (2020): World Economic Outlook Update, June, (https://www.imf.org/en/Publications/WEO/Issues/2020/06/24/WEOUpdateJune2020), accessed on November 6, 2020.

Economics, the global economic forecasting firm.[82] Reportedly, even Bangladesh's fiscal support is over 2 per cent of GDP.

Chart 2: Country fiscal measures in response to the COVID-19 pandemic

Countries are providing sizable fiscal support through budgetary measures, as well as off-budget liquidity.

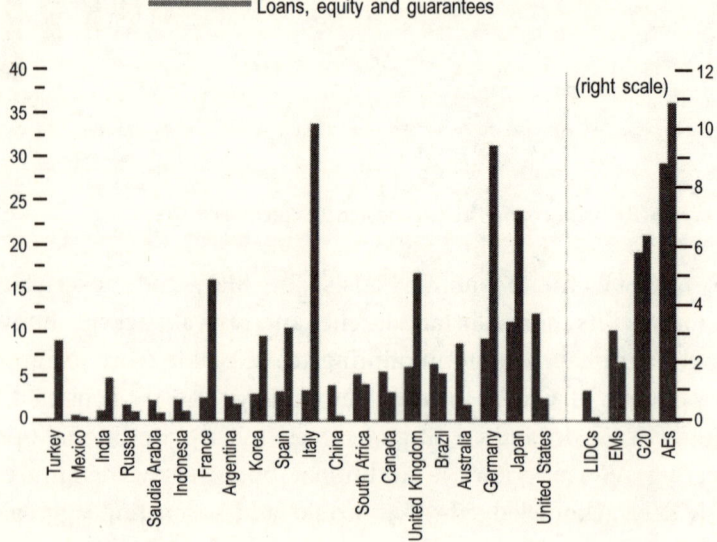

Source: IMF, 2020

---

[82]Oxford Economics's report titled *A Reopening Gone Wrong* by Priyanka Kishore, the head of India and Southeast Asia Economics, in an interview with the online magazine rediff.com (https://www.rediff.com/business/interview/it-will-take-longest-for-indias-growth-to-return/20200810.htm) accessed on November 6, 2020

Thus, many countries have suspended fiscal deficit and public debt targets for now. As the IMF report said[83]:

> The steep contraction in output and ensuing fall in revenues, along with sizable discretionary support, have led to a surge in government debt and deficits. [...] global public debt is expected to reach an all-time high, exceeding 101 per cent of GDP in 2020–21—a surge of 19 percentage points from a year ago. Meanwhile, the average overall fiscal deficit is expected to soar to 14 per cent of GDP in 2020, 10 percentage points higher than last year.

What to Do Now?

Our suggestions have three parts: (a) minimize the adverse health outcomes, and restore jobs and livelihoods; (b) double public health expenditure in three years on a mission mode; and (c) revive fixed investment growth in industry and infrastructure. The following two sections offer the details.

The immediate tasks are to (a) control the pandemic by sustained emergency public facilities in smaller towns and rural areas where the virus seems to be spreading rapidly, and (b) restore output, incomes and livelihoods to the last year's level by the next FY, 2021. As the domestic output has contracted more than previously anticipated, another dose of fiscal stimulus is called for, focussed on boosting public spending—a view the IMF has also advocated.

Allocations made in May 2020 seem to have exhausted substantially in rural areas by early September, indicating the dire unemployment situation (as per news reports)[84]; hence, a need to

---

[83]IMF (2020): World Economic Outlook Update, June 2020, International Monetary Fund, Washington DC. p.17.
[84]Sumedha Pal. (September 11, 2020). Budgetary Allocation Exhausted, COVID-19 Package Not Released Yet: NREGA Tracker, Newsclick. Accessed

replenish resources for employment generation programmes. Free food distribution and public distribution system (PDS) allocations perhaps need to be supplemented to avoid the health pandemic turning into a hunger and nutritional crisis.

Good kharif sowing is expectedly generating on-farm jobs, reducing the demand for rural employment programmes and food distribution. But there is no reason for withdrawing public action anytime soon.

As the health pandemic is here for a while (as experts indicate), the government needs to prepare a medium-term strategy to double public health expenditure to 2.6 per cent of GDP by 2024–25. India perhaps needs a public health revolution of the kind the advanced countries underwent during the late nineteenth and early twentieth centuries to control infectious diseases, as Monica Dasgupta's research demonstrated.[85] Such a strategic plan would call for investment in urban drainage, sanitation and drinking water. Since building such physical facilities are labour-intensive, using local resources would boost employment of unskilled labour. Jean Drèze's idea of Decentralised Urban Employment and Training could be the scheme for building public health infrastructure using an urban employment guarantee programme.[86] The government could aggressively tap into the special lending windows, now available with multilateral funding agencies, to cope with the pandemic. They could provide low-cost budgetary resources, and also offer technical assistance for augmenting public health capabilities, which are now very poor at the state and local levels.

---

at https://www.newsclick.in/Budgetary-Allocation-Exhausted-COVID-19-Package-Released-NREGA-Tracker, on 6 November 2020.

[85] Monica Das Gupta (2005): Public Health in India: An Overview. Policy Research Working Paper; No. 3787, the World Bank, Washington, DC.

[86] J. Drèze (2020, September 10). An Indian Duet For Urban Jobs. Retrieved November 02, 2020, from https://www.bloombergquint.com/opinion/an-indian-duet-for-urban-jobs

Beyond the restoration and rehabilitation, economic growth needs to revive urgently. During the last decade (i.e., the 2010s), the most significant contributor to the economic slowdown was fixed investment rate as a proportion of GDP. India's investment rate has declined by close to 10 percentage points of GDP from its peak of 38–39 per cent attained in 2008–09, which is an unprecedented collapse.

Export growth also fell, but net exports, as a proportion of GDP, declined marginally as the oil import bill came down precipitously. With global economic contraction and the cracks in the multilateral trading agreement, India cannot be hopeful about export revival anytime soon. The large domestic market is an advantage. Atmanirbharta also calls for a rising share of local value addition by firms owned and controlled by Indian nationals.

Growth should avoid—learning from the recent experience—predation of the rural and informal economy (by indiscriminate deregulation of mining and environmental laws, as seems likely from the recent regulatory reforms). Nor should it favour crony capitalists, or 'Bollygarchs'—to use James Crabtree's picturesque phrase to allude to politically connected conglomerates. Moreover, India needs an ambitious investment plan if the government is still serious about the PM's aspirational target of a $5 trillion economy by 2024–25, announced last year.

Make in India, initiated in 2014, was intended to raise the manufacturing sector's share in GDP to 25 per cent (from 14–15 per cent at the time), and creating 100 million additional jobs in the industry by 2021–22. Five years on, manufacturing output growth has plummeted, leading to the loss of 3.5 million jobs between 2011–12 and 2017–18. The government frittered away its energies seeking to improve the country's global ranking in the World Bank's questionable index of Ease of Doing Business.[87]

---

[87] R. Nagaraj. (2019). 'Make in India: Why Didn't the Lion Roar?', *The India*

The rank did move up impressively, but miserably failed to boost the industrial economy.

The pandemic and the low-intensity border dispute with China since June 2020 are a rude reminder of how vulnerable India has become to imports.[88] The Make in India initiative, therefore, needs a serious reimagination. It is worth recalling how Maruti in 1982 triggered the modernization of India's automotive industry, or how the Oil and Natural Gas Corporation helped overcome import dependence on oil by quickly developing the Bombay High offshore fields after the second Oil Shock in 1979, spurring an industrial revival in the 1980s.

Recent case studies of small firm clusters in manufacturing across the country have brought to light how the infrastructure and state support at the ground level appeared frozen in times of the pre-reform era, despite changes in definitions and terminology. Such clusters—mostly producing labour-intensive goods—seem to cry out for public support. There are compelling examples of how some clusters had stood up to the global competition when reasonable government assistance came forward.[89]

If Make in India and Atmanirbhar Bharat are about overcoming technological stagnation, India has to step up R&D expenditure. Here is a telling comparison with China. Chart 3 shows R&D expenditure as a proportion of GDP in India and China between 1996 and 2018.

Until 1999, the expenditure ratios in the two countries were identical, at 0.8 per cent of GDP. Over the next 20 years, for China, the proportion nearly trebled to 2.2 per cent of GDP. For

---

Forum, April 13.
[88]Biswajit Dhar and K.S. Chalapati Rao (2020): India's Economic Dependence on China, *The India Forum*, August 7.
[89]R. Nagaraj. (2021) (edited). *Industrialisation for Employment and Growth in India: Lessons from Small Firm Clusters and Beyond*, Cambridge University Press (Forthcoming).

India, the ratio declined to 0.6 per cent by 2018. The divergence is incredibly sharp after the 2008 global financial crisis. Considering that China's GDP has grown at a faster rate in this period, the gap in the absolute size of resources invested in scientific research is enormous.

Chart 3: R&D expenditure as % of GDP, India and China

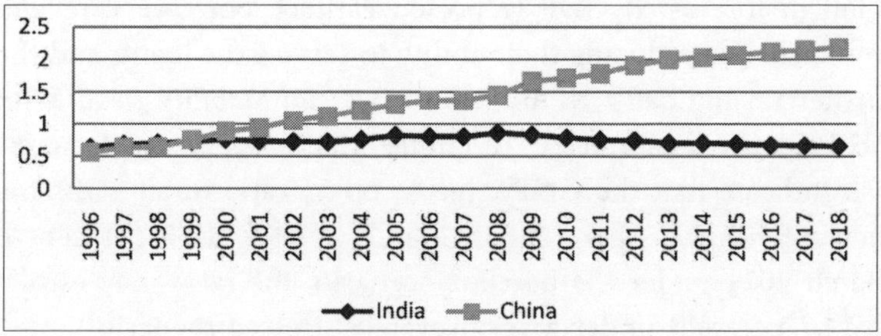

Source: World Bank, World Development Indicators

To forge the above ideas into a credible and consistent strategy, India needs an industrial policy, with suitable instruments for execution. To finance it, reinvent development banks to provide long-term credit, that is, beyond the five-year term the commercial banks currently offer. History shows that no Asian economy has been industrialized—from Japan to China—without a state-led industrialization strategy and development banks to support it. China, despite its rhetoric of globalization and market reforms since Deng Xiaoping opened up the economy in 1978, never took its eyes off industrial policy and development banks underpinning the national goals.

Financing the Growth Plan

The preceding suggestions appear like a wish list indeed. Many may endorse these ideas. The challenge though is to find real, i.e., non-inflationary, resources to finance the investments. Here are a few ideas, though detailed budgetary arithmetic is beyond the scope of the essay.

The private corporate sector—the engine of the Dream Run during the 2000s—is not up to the task now, with mounting debt and declining profitability. The banking sector that fuelled the growth with copious credit is now neck-deep in NPAs. With a fall in forecasted GDP (reported earlier), borrowers' revenue would shrink, reducing their ability to service the loans, and thus further raising bank NPAs. RBI's *Financial Stability Report*, July 2020, admitted as much.[90] To quote: 'Macro stress tests for credit risk indicate that the GNPA [gross NPA] ratio of all SCBs may increase from 8.5 per cent in March 2020 to 12.5 per cent by March 2021 under the baseline scenario; the ratio may escalate to 14.7 per cent under a very severely stressed scenario.'

To expect foreign capital to fill in the investment gap is wishful thinking. To illustrate, at the peak of the boom of 2003–08, when the economy was ticking at close to 9 per cent annually, FDI inflow was at best 2–2.5 per cent of GDP. In China, FDI inflow never exceeded 5 per cent of GDP, most of which was anyway domestic capital round-tripped via Hong Kong to secure better property rights.

History shows—without exception—that economies that have successfully industrialized have relied mostly on domestic savings. Foreign capital could be a catalyst bringing in technology, promoting 'learning by doing' and to secure access to developed markets via global buying agents or supply chains. To attract greenfield FDI, the host country needs to provide the complementary social and physical infrastructure, which, as known, is woefully lacking. Hence India has to invest massively in infrastructure of the kind noted above.

---

[90]RBI press release on the *Financial Stability Report*, July 2020

More seriously, history also demonstrates that no modern nation can hope to become 'atmanirbhar', or self-reliant, by relying mainly on foreign capital and technology, whose risk-adjusted costs tend to be high.

That leaves us with public investment and strategically significant public sector enterprises. Mobilizing public expenditure in recessionary times, as a counter-cyclical policy, is a well-accepted principle in economics since Keynes. With little demand for credit forthcoming from the private sector and declining interest rates close to zero in real terms (known as the 'zero lower bound'), a national development bank can be an instrument for mobilizing capital from the market. Such resources can be productively used in projects with a high rate of return, such as social and economic infrastructure. Such investments are unlikely to 'crowd out' private investment, and instead could bring in complementary private investment[91]—as recent experience indicates.

It is perhaps worth recollecting the NDA government's experience in 1999–2000. Faced with a decelerating GDP growth rate and industrial production after the Asian Financial Crisis in 1997, the Vajpayee government launched two major investment projects. One was the Golden Quadrilateral road reconstruction programme to connect metro cities with high-quality roads; and the second was the Pradhan Mantri Gram Sadak Yojana to construct all-weather roads to connect villages and hamlets with a population of 500 people or above. These public investments ushered in the automobile revolution, boosting output growth.[92] Such massive labour-intensive projects offered an alternative employment opportunity for rural workers, contributing to a rise

---

[91] R. Nagaraj. (2017). 'Economic Reforms and Manufacturing Sector Growth: Need for Reconfiguring the Industrialisation Model', *Economic and Political Weekly*, Vol. 52, No. 2, January 14.
[92] R. Nagaraj. (2013). 'The Dream Run: 2003-08: Understanding the Recent Boom and its Aftermath', *Economic and Political Weekly*, Vol. 48, May 18.

in real rural wages—probably for a first in post-independence India.

However, in the mainstream economic theory and popular media, such evidence goes against the tenets of fiscal virtue. Financial markets, it is argued, are expected to 'punish' such fiscal indulgence triggering capital flight, potentially precipitating macroeconomic crises. The underlying reasoning is as follows: rising public expenditure could lead to breaching fiscal deficit, increasing public debt-to-GDP ratio. The rising fiscal deficit could stoke inflation fears and BoP deficit, potentially causing macroeconomic instability, downgrading the credit rating and raising the cost of external borrowing.

The preceding line of reasoning is possible when aggregate demand seriously overshoots aggregate supply, calling for macroeconomic stabilization. The current situation is, however, different: It is one of inadequate aggregate demand as the economy is operating below the full-employment output. As the private sector is unable to use the additional credit at any interest rate due to the elevated debt burden, rising public spending is unlikely to pre-empt private investment. Government expenditure, on the contrary, could stimulate demand from the private sector and thus augment output growth. Further, if such public investments help relieve critical supply constraints—such as roads or ports or electricity—chances of public expenditure leading to inflation and external imbalance are, in principle, remote. Hence, what matters is not the expansion of public spending *per se*, but its productivity.

In 2013, in the context of weak output growth in the US, despite interest rates being close to zero, Robert Solow, the Nobel Laureate, writing in *The New York Times*, said:

> '... *in bad times like now, Treasury bonds are not squeezing finance for investment out of the market.* On the contrary, debt-financed

government spending adds to the demand for privately produced goods and services, and the bonds provide a home for excess savings. When employment returns to normal, we can return to debt reduction' [*emphasis in original*].[93]

Beyond borrowing from the bond market, the government could also borrow directly from the central bank (RBI in India), which is known as debt monetization, or deficit financing. Operationally, it was earlier known as RBI's 'ways and means' advance to the central government. As deficit financing was reportedly the source of fiscal profligacy and inflation, the practice ended in 1997, as per a formal agreement between the government and the RBI.

However, given the current unprecedented situation of output contraction, there is a case for reviving the practice, if temporarily, to augment the government's resources. Extraordinary times call for such unconventional measures—just as the US Federal Reserve-devised 'Quantitative Easing' (QE) after the 2008 financial crisis. QE provided cash to Wall Street conglomerates by buying up government securities to reduce interest rates and induce banks to lend to the private sector. Likewise, now, one many argue, why not extend the same principle to put money in the hands of the government to boost public spending to save jobs and growth or provide UBI by putting money directly in people's hands?[94]

Many countries are doing it, as the IMF report quoted earlier showed. For example, the UK's ruling Conservative government has reintroduced 'ways and means' borrowing from the Treasury to support small firms. It is akin to restoring ways and means advances from the RBI in India.

Thus, there is now a case for monetization of public debt,

---

[93]Robert Solow. (2013). 'Our Debt, Ourselves'. *The New York Times*, February 27.
[94]Frances Coppola. (2019). *The Case for People's Quantitative Easing*, Polity Press.

subject to inflation. If the preceding arguments are accepted in principle, preparing an action plan could follow, fleshing out many policy suggestions made in the essay.

Structural Reforms Can Wait, for Now

Structural reforms are meant to reduce government intervention in various markets to augment the supply of output. In theory, they yield results in the medium term, when excessive state regulations are supposedly throttling output growth.[95] In the post-COVID situation, as shown earlier, output growth is constrained for lack of aggregate demand, not of supply. Hence, the structural reforms are unlikely to boost output growth now. Admittedly, there are lockdown-induced transport and labour supply bottlenecks; they are temporary.

The government is preoccupied with structural reforms, however. Most of the Atmanirbhar Bharat economic stimulus, as widely acknowledged, consisted of easing supply constraints. The government seems to seldom miss an opportunity to introduce structural reforms, ignoring the need of the hour. For instance, at the peak of the health pandemic, many state governments sought to practically do away with the labour laws. Trade union federations have unanimously opposed the dilutions: ILO has rebuked such measures as they go against the ILO charter (to which India is a signatory), and the high courts have dismissed many such ordinances. Ostensibly, reasons for the legal changes are to attract foreign investors seeking to move out of China, given the growing geopolitical tensions in global trade. However, what the state governments failed to realize is that the scrapping of the labour laws amid the lockdown may further reduce employment

---

[95]For a formal definition of structural reforms, see European Central Bank's explainers. https://www.ecb.europa.eu/explainers/tell-me/html/what-are-structural_reforms.en.html

and hence reduce aggregate demand and hurt the prospects of economic recovery.

Similarly, the government also sought to eliminate misuse of bogus ration cards by introducing the 'one-country, one ration card' scheme. While the leakages of PDS indeed needed to be plugged, the ongoing livelihood crisis is the least opportune moment for it, as the reform measure could potentially deny foodgrain access to the poor, and could accentuate hunger and malnutrition in distressful times.

The long-term binding constraints on stepping up India's aggregate output growth were food, fuel (i.e., imported oil) and foreign exchange. We have none of these constraints now, with overflowing foodgrain stocks (and an expected bumper crop this year), historically low oil prices in real terms and burgeoning foreign exchange reserves (by capital inflows, not from export surplus).

Conclusion

The COVID-19 pandemic, and the lockdown to contain it, have made everyday life difficult and unpredictable, especially for the poor and unemployed. GDP in absolute terms during April–June 2020 shrunk by 24 per cent, compared to the same period the previous year. FY20 is forecasted to end with the economy shrinking by 10.3 per cent, compared to the previous year, as per IMF WEO October 2020. The output contraction comes on top of a prolonged economic slowdown, at least since 2014–15. Muddied official data, however, fails to adequately capture the ground reality. Low output growth has raised UR%, reduced per capita consumption and increased the proportion of the population in absolute poverty.

The post-COVID-19 economic policy should have three distinct components: (i) quickly restoring jobs and livelihoods,

(ii) implementing an emergency medium-term plan to double public health expenditure to face any eventuality of the spreading pandemic, and (iii) boost investment demand to revive economic growth to 7–8 per cent per year to create gainful employment and reduce absolute poverty. Structural reforms intended to ease supply constraints (supposedly by dysfunctional state interventions) can wait for now, as there are no significant supply shortages in the aggregate (beyond the lockdown-induced disruptions).

Restoring jobs and livelihoods would call for boosting current government expenditure, including massive public works programmes both in urban and rural areas, and income support. A public health emergency plan can be tied up with a public works programme in urban areas. The government could tap into emergency funds by multilateral agencies to fight the pandemic.

The task of reviving investment demand would have to rest with the public sector and its enterprises. With private corporate sector in no position to step up investment on account of debt and commercial banks mired in mounting NPAs, public infrastructure investment—financed by public debt, including deficit financing (subject to inflation)—is the only credible option now. Even to attract foreign investment in manufacturing—as part of the Make in India initiative—a complementary infrastructure investment is necessary, which has to mostly come from the public sector. Such investments also function as a signalling device for foreign capital to show the national commitment to promote manufacturing.

The pandemic and border skirmishes with China since June have exposed India's rising import dependence and technological stagnancy. India needs to design a new industrial policy and set up a development bank to provide long-term credit that is currently not available. To make India atmanirbhar, the objective of Make in India should be to make primarily *for* India for now, using increasingly domestic capital, enterprise and technology.

To finance the post-COVID industrial strategy, as in many countries, India needs to shed its fiscal orthodoxy and embrace an expansionary budgetary stance. It should include public debt monetization for a while, subject only to inflationary threat. With no significant supply constraints on the horizon, structural reforms can be set aside for now.

◆

R. Nagaraj was a professor at the Indira Gandhi Institute of Development Research, Mumbai. His most recent work is an edited volume called *Industrialisation for Employment and Growth in India: Lessons from Small Firm Clusters and Beyond*, to be published by Cambridge University Press.

NEW THREATS TO PAID EMPLOYMENT OF WOMEN

A.V. Jose[96]

There is a predicament facing women all over India, manifested through low work participation arising from non-availability of jobs, a professed preference for regular jobs, and a willingness and availability to work longer hours. These are precisely the conditions that cause a further deterioration of wages and work conditions, leading to what some analysts would call a market-clearing situation. The COVID-19 pandemic now gripping the country has made the situation worse for women's employment. Updates on the employment situation in the lockdown period suggest a drastic reduction of work participation, severely affecting the employment of young workers and women.[97]

Countering any downward slide in wage/salary levels and working conditions ought to figure prominently in the public policy design. Perhaps it is time to try new and innovative approaches to employment promotion, which require a prudent combination of market interventions. Post-COVID public policy

---

[96]The author wishes to pay respect to the memory of two eminent analysts of the Indian economy, Professors A. Vaidyanathan and N. Krishnaji, who passed away recently. They pioneered many insightful studies on land distribution and labour utilization in India. He has drawn from their works without attributing any responsibility on them for his interpretation.

[97]Mahesh Vyas. (2020). Weekly columns in *Business Standard* on employment in India, using sample survey data of CMIE.

must focus specifically on how more women could take up paid employment.

Data on work participation among women in Indian states show that participation rates are extremely low, but the URs% are very high. We discuss here the LFPR-W and the worker population rate of women (WPR-W) for the whole of India, based on the Periodic Labour Force Survey (PLFS) estimates for 2018–19, while exploring some determinants of women's employment.

As a first step in understanding the problem, we need to sort out some issues concerning the measurement of employment and unemployment. There are two measures of employment used intermittently in the Indian context. One is the LFPR, which takes the employed and the unemployed together as a share of the working-age population (15-plus years). The second is the worker-population ratio, which takes only the employed as a share of the working-age population.

There are two methods used in sample surveys to estimate the number of workers. One is the 'usual status' approach, which identifies a worker in the labour force either as employed or unemployed during the preceding year, depending on what they 'usually' did. The workers who have worked and/or have been looking for work for more than six months of the year are in the usual principal status. Those who have worked or have been looking for work for more than a month in the past year are in the subsidiary status. A second approach is to identify a person either as employed or unemployed over the preceding week. This is her current weekly status (CWS). The PLFS, which commenced in 2017, leans more on the CWS approach. It has the advantage of a shorter recall period and conforms to standard international practices.

Puzzle of Low Work Participation

The first puzzle is why so few women in India are doing remunerative work when by 'work', we mean economic activities that 'qualify' as employment over and above what women do as caregivers at home. The LFPR-W in India is among the lowest in the world. Within the working-age group of 15-plus years, the rate in India is just 22 per cent, 23 per cent in rural areas and a still lower 20 per cent in urban areas.[98] Comparable estimates for other countries are close to 60 per cent in the nations of Europe and well above 60 per cent in East Asia, notably China.[99] On the other hand, the proportion of male workers in India is not strikingly different from the rest of the world.[100]

We come across two patterns, which stand out in defiance of the logic of economic development. First, ordinarily we would expect transformative changes in developing countries to bring at least some increase in the presence of women in paid work. This has not happened in India, where the participation of women in the labour force continues to remain low. Second, and equally importantly, urbanization has not precipitated any visible increase in women's work participation.

Historically, in most parts of India, women's participation in work outside the household has remained low, a phenomenon that probably has roots in the practice of settled agriculture in South Asia. Intensive farming of field crops, as it evolved in India, relied more on the use of draught animals and human labour,

---

[98] PLFS. (2020). *Annual Report of the Periodic Labour Force Survey*, 2018–19, Ministry of Statistics and Programme Implementation, Government of India. A-217.

[99] The comparative estimates are available in the *Year Book of Labour Statistics*, an online publication of the International Labour Organisation.

[100] The LFPR of men in India is 76 per cent, 69 per cent in OECD countries, 77 per cent in South Asia and 76 per cent in East Asia, according to the ILO's *Year Book of Labour Statistics*.

the latter forcibly extracted from the subordinate sub-castes of society.[101] Men and women of labour households, mostly at the lower end of a caste hierarchy and kept at the subsistence margin, were commandeered for farm operations outside their homes.[102] Ester Boserup had noted that as the cropping pattern shifted in India from long fallow to short fallow and more intensive cropping, the women of land-holding households withdrew from subsistence farming, with rising productivity of land and labour, and engaged themselves in unpaid work.[103]

The pattern remained unchanged for many centuries. Women not doing physical work outside the household was considered a mark of prestige and economic status. This naturally got reflected in India's work participation rates, as revealed in various censuses and National Sample Surveys of the old NSSO. An extreme example is in the state of Bihar from the Gangetic plains, where the LFPR-W in the working-age groups even today is only 4 per cent against the all-India average of 22 per cent.[104] One cannot help surmise that the past several decades of development have not been accompanied by any substantial increase in women's work participation, neither in Bihar nor in the rest of India.

Quite possibly, the organization of agriculture on extensive landholdings in some parts of the country has led to increased hiring of women in agricultural operations. The pauperization of peasant households, which Krishnaji drew attention to, could have

---

[101]A. Vaidyanathan. (1978). *Labour absorption in Indian agriculture: Some exploratory investigations*, (Bangkok: ILO-ARTEP).

[102]Dharma Kumar. (1965). *Land and Caste in South India: Agricultural Labour in the Madras Presidency during the Nineteenth Century*, (Cambridge: Cambridge University Press).

[103]Ester Boserup. (1965). *The Conditions of Agricultural Growth*. (New York: Aldine Publishing Company).

[104]PLFS. (2020). *Annual Report of the Periodic Labour Force Survey*, 2018-19, Ministry of Statistics and Programme Implementation, Government of India. A-217.

contributed towards the wage labour for commercial farming.[105] Such hiring was, however, not sufficient to bring about any tangible improvement of the LFPR-W. This is now a maximum of 35 per cent in one or two states, but in most, it is far below this level.[106]

Ordinarily, we would expect urbanization, to the extent it has happened, to have positively influenced the entry of women into the labour force. This is not the case in most Indian states. As we noted earlier, the LFPR-W is lower in urban areas than in rural areas. This is contrary to the experience of the industrialized world. An inference drawn is that currently there are no pull factors, offering decent employment opportunities for women in the cities. If the urban enclaves of India are not acting as magnets to draw more women into paid employment, the question naturally arises as to whether current policies are appropriate for promotion of women's employment and income-earning opportunities for them. Probably not. There is, therefore, a compelling case to rethink the strategies towards the goal.

One redeeming feature of urban India is a positive association between the usual status LFPR-W and the monthly per capita consumption expenditure of households. As we move up the decile classes of consumption expenditure, the work participation of women increases, though at a slow pace. It implies that women work and contribute positively to the income of their households. This observation is valid for rural households, too, but the scale of women's involvement is lower than in urban areas.[107]

---

[105] N. Krishnaji. (1992). *Pauperising Agriculture*, Sameeksha Trust (Bombay: Oxford University Press)

[106] PLFS. (2020). *Annual Report of the Periodic Labour Force Survey*, 2018-19, Ministry of Statistics and Programme Implementation, Government of India. A-217.

[107] Ibid. A-182, 185

Another feature is a positive association between the usual status LFPR-W and the educational qualifications of women, from higher secondary school onwards. Educational accomplishments are essential determinants of women's employment and of their household income levels. For instance, in both the urban and rural areas of Kerala, the participation rate is 47 per cent among graduates, 78 per cent among postgraduate and 52 per cent among those with certificates or diplomas of specific occupations. The corresponding all-India averages are lower, but follow a similar pattern.[108] This suggests that in conformity with a universal trend, education leads to greater participation of women in the skilled categories of work. But there is a caveat: they take up jobs only if they are available and accessible.

The downside of a positive association between LFPR-W and higher education is that the UR% becomes higher as women move up the education ladder. To understand this better, one can look at the figures based on the usual status of the working-age groups, both in rural and urban areas. These show that unemployment is conspicuously higher among educated women than men. From the higher secondary level onwards, the UR% of women is at least 50 per cent or more, even twice the corresponding ratio for men.[109] For instance, among graduate women, in 2018–19 it was 25 per cent and among the postgraduate, 24 per cent. The average rates for men in a similar setting were 15 per cent and 11 per cent, respectively.[110] The figures suggest that any advancement of women's schooling is likely to be accompanied by a higher incidence of unemployment among them, unless, of course, more jobs are created.

---

[108]Ibid., A-127.
[109]Ibid., A-145.
[110]Ibid., A-144.

Possible Policy Interventions

The upshot of the argument is that any Indian state making progress with the education of women would face problems in absorbing the educated into the workforce. It is not just a frictional or transitory problem that is likely to pass when the economy attains faster growth. Here is a structural problem that requires policy interventions by the state and all the social actors concerned. How do we go about it? Some evidence gathered from the PLFS facilitates a discussion of possible policy interventions.

First, let's take a look at the distribution of women workers in different status categories of employment. There is a higher concentration of women workers in the category of regular wage/salary earners than in other groups such as self-employed or casual wage labour. In urban areas, 57 per cent of all women were engaged in regular wage/salary employment against 33 per cent in self-employment and 9 per cent in casual labour.[111] Most women workers in the cities would rather wait, if they can afford to, for regular jobs than do other kinds of work. One compelling reason for their preference for regular employment is the prevalence of wide differentials in earnings across status groups. Table 1, compiled from the PLFS, gives a profile of such differentials for the whole of India.

The average monthly earnings of men and women in different status groups elicit some notable observations.[112] One, the earnings of women with regular jobs were more than twice the earnings from self-employment or casual work, both in rural and urban areas. Second, the rural–urban disparity in earnings remains pervasive in each status group, but is less severe among regular

---

[111] Ibid., A-230.

[112] The table gives the simple average of earnings of the three status groups reported in four quarters of the PLFS. As for casual labour, the daily wage rates were multiplied by the days worked per month, derived from PLFS Table 45.

TABLE 1
Average earnings per month of workers in different status categories of employment and some associated ratios, all India, 2018–19

	Rural		Urban	
	Men	Women	Men	Women
Earnings (₹) per month				
Regular Wage/Salary Earners	13,549	8,724	19,199	14,843
Self Employed	9,420	4,216	16,725	6,612
Casual Labour	6,831	3,999	8,117	5,059
Ratio of earnings as %				
Self Employed/Regular Wage Earners	69.53	48.32	87.11	44.55
Casual Labour/Regular Wage Earners	50.42	45.83	42.28	34.08
Women's Earnings as % of Men's				
Regular Wage/Salary Earner	–	64.39	–	77.31
Self Employed	–	44.75	–	39.54
Casual Labour	–	58.54	–	62.32

Source: PLFS (2018-19, Tables 42–45)

employees in urban areas. More importantly, the gender gap in income is conspicuous both in rural and urban areas; women earn less than half that of men in self-employment and less than two-thirds in casual work. The disparity is less for regular workers, especially in urban areas, where women receive about 80 per cent of men's earnings. These factors add to the attraction of steady jobs, which women prefer, whether or not they move to urban areas.

There is a severe shortage of regular jobs in urban areas. Industry-wise, less than 30 per cent of women workers are engaged in manufacturing jobs, and the rest (65 per cent) are in the service industries, where education and skill content are essential criteria for employment.[113] One point to emphasize is that urban women with regular jobs work more hours per week compared to women in self-employment or casual work. Also, a small, but not an insignificant proportion of them (more than twice that of men), expressed their willingness and availability to work for more hours. The evidence points to the labour-intensive nature of operations in urban areas, where women tend to be underpaid even as they take up regular jobs.

The focus is on making work more attractive to the 'potentially employed', a category that covers the unemployed and those outside the labour force. They broadly belong to two categories: the less skilled, prone to doing casual wage labour; and the better skilled, currently on the sidelines waiting for the right offers and placements. Both categories include the discouraged women workers, who would naturally expect the rewards from paid work outside the household to exceed their opportunity cost or the reservation price. This would be roughly equivalent to the income generated directly and indirectly through numerous household-centred activities. Quite possibly, the combined value of wages and benefits from work outside, currently on offer in most states, especially in urban areas, is less than the reservation price. One option is to make paid work more attractive by raising the returns to meet the aspirations of potential women workers. A better package of minimum wages and social security benefits addressed to different tiers and skill categories of the labour force and made accessible to all women can make a vast difference to the present employment situation.

A two-pronged approach—one to raise the floor wage as a

---

[113]PLFS. (2020). *Annual Report of the Periodic Labour Force Survey*, 2018–19, Ministry of Statistics and Programme Implementation, Government of India. A-224.

component of the reservation price in any state or region, and the other to enhance the content of social security benefits of workers—can have an impact on employment outcomes.[114] The first is primarily addressed to the less-skilled workers, women in particular. The floor wage itself depends on a basket of entitlements, including food, nutrition, shelter, education, health and civic amenities, which the workers gain access to as the essentials of a dignified life for all citizens. It depends on the scale and content of social spending on the basic needs prevalent in any state. There is enough evidence from the developing countries to argue that social spending with a redistributive thrust helps to set a solid floor, below which wages will not fall due to downward pressure from the supply side. A socially engineered minimum wage, supported through public expenditure, can safeguard low-income groups against any distress-driven migration. More importantly, it can help them cross the barriers to entry in urban labour markets and empower them to navigate towards skill mobility and remunerative jobs.

The second component concerns the strengthening of institutional safeguards for social security as a practical way of drawing more skilled women into paid employment. The thrust of state interventions should be to encourage all workers—in particular, women—to pursue their aspirations for a secure and healthy living during and beyond their working lives. It is an eminently feasible goal, gaining legitimacy and traction in many developing countries that have crossed the low-income threshold.

A compelling reason for policy intervention for social security is that people who are about to retire have, ahead of them, longer lives without disability. However, there are some prerequisites for attaining the goal of universal social security. First and foremost,

---

[114]The ensuing discussion on the two components of public policy is also outlined in A.V. Jose. (2019). 'Changing Structure of Employment in Indian States' Working Paper 478, Centre for Development Studies, Thiruvananthapuram.

enhance the reach of social insurance programmes, so that all workers can build their individually owned nest eggs through provident funds, pension annuities and health schemes using contributions from their employers as well as by themselves (as employees and the self-employed).

Many emerging economies are taking the lead in building annuities for all workers earning regular incomes, which eventually become income streams for pensions and healthcare. They follow a maxim that whenever a worker gets hired on a regular paid job, pro-rata the employer bears the cost of his/her retirement pension and healthcare. The state specifies the scale of contribution based on the workers' earnings, which would mature into annuities for liquidation at the time of retirement. At the same time, for casual workers without a regular income, public policy envisages the creation of means-tested social assistance, giving them access to public provisioning of old-age pensions and health services. Such schemes are beginning to operate in India under the National Pension Schemes and the Prime Minister Suraksha Bima Yojana. They have the potential to build on the social security entitlements of all workers, in particular those with low earnings.

In India, there is abundant scope for fine-tuning the existing institutions for raising the floor wages and enhancing the reach of social security, so that they can take on more responsibilities for the well-being of all workers. The first is meant to encourage more work participation of women and the second, to offer a better deal to skilled workers. What is needed at this stage is a broad-based dialogue involving the practitioners of labour policy on the means of creating appropriate institutions to safeguard the entitlements of workers, women in particular, and make them equal partners in the society.

Conclusion

Against this grim picture of women's employment in India, the sharp decline in economic activity due to the COVID pandemic and the lockdown has only made the situation worse. The country needs imaginative labour policies for the promotion of women's employment in the non-farm sectors. Governments at the Centre and in the states have to play a supportive role in drawing more women, especially the discouraged workers, into paid work. Public policy interventions can make work more attractive by offering higher floor wages to the less skilled and improved social security benefits to the better skilled. There is room for building a support system that can improve work participation and work-related benefits for all women in India.

◆

A.V. Jose has been on the staff of the Centre for Development Studies, Thiruvananthapuram, and the International Labour Organisation, Geneva. He was the director of Gulati Institute of Finance and Taxation (GIFT), Thiruvananthapuram, and is presently an honorary fellow at GIFT.

PANDEMIC AND MIGRANTS: MISSED OPPORTUNITIES AND THE ROAD AHEAD

S. Irudaya Rajan

The COVID-19 pandemic crisis, ever since its beginnings in late 2019 in China, has travelled to over 200 countries and infected over 40 million people around the globe, a count that is rising daily even after a year of its onset. The pandemic, an unprecedented episode in the history of the globalized world, saw a shutdown of not only economies, but also human mobility. And while the economic shutdown has been reversed, human mobility remains restricted within and among countries. Though the larger effects of the lockdown of the economy are yet to be completely understood, its effects on one group of persons were immediately seen. The migrants felt the strain of the lockdown as it impacted not only their lives and livelihoods, but also their mobility—a reality that reared its ugly head in the days immediately after the lockdown, which saw tragic scenes of migrants leaving their places of work in the most inhospitable conditions and often on foot. This led to tragic outcomes of desperation, homelessness and numerous cases of migrant deaths.[115] Even the plight of millions of international migrants came to the fore, with a number of

---

[115] A. Banerji. (2020). Nearly 200 migrant workers killed on India's roads during coronavirus lockdown. *Reuters*. https://www.reuters.com/article/us-health-coronavirus-india-migrants/nearly-200-migrant-workers-killed-on-indias-roads-during-coronavirus-lockdown-idUSKBN2392LG

them being forced to come back due to loss of livelihoods at their places of work.[116]

India's Migrants

The 2011 Indian Census enumerated 453.6 million as migrants, based on place of last residence—an increase of 139 million migrants from 314.5 million in 2001. In the absence of a reliable estimate, the number of internal migrants can be estimated to be around 600 million (Chart 1), based on earlier trends.

Chart 1: Trends of internal migration in India, 1971–2021

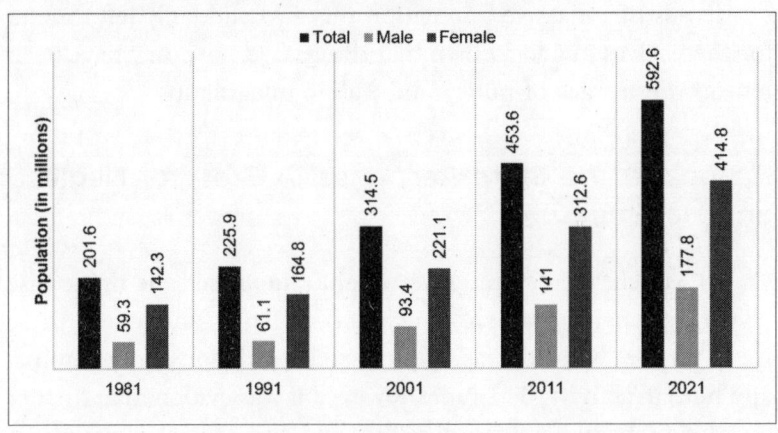

Source: Based on Indian Censuses (1971–2011) and my projections

Out of 600 million migrants, one-third of them are inter-state and inter-district migrants—200 million. Among them, two-

---

[116]V.K. George. (2020). Indian labourers abroad are in dire need of help, say experts. *The Hindu*. Retrieved from: thehindu.com/news/national/coronavirus-indian-labourers-in-gcc-countries-are-in-dire-need-of-help-say-migration-experts-irudaya-rajan-and-ginu-zacharaia-oommen/article31318501.ece

thirds (140 million) are estimated to be migrant workers.[117] Migrants are mainly concentrated in temporary, informal and casual employment, and are most vulnerable to exploitation.

On the other hand, India has over 20 million migrants abroad. Among them, 10 million live in the six Gulf Cooperation Council (GCC) countries of Saudi Arabia, United Arab Emirates, Qatar, Kuwait, Oman and Bahrain. Most of these workers are unskilled and semi-skilled, working in the construction and other labour-intensive sectors, and contribute equally in terms of remittances, with India receiving $83 billion in 2019.[118] A lot of these migrants lost their jobs and were held up in precarious conditions in their places of work, having to be evacuated through special missions.

It was this massive population that was suddenly left to fend for themselves in a lockdown that showcased how they have been left on the fringes of policy and public imagination.

A Look at the State Response: A Story of Neglect and Half-measures

On 24 March, the central government announced the first phase of the national lockdown, which subsequently underwent three more phases, with increasingly relaxed regulations on economic and human activity. By 7 June, however, it was evident that further lockdowns would not be possible, and the central government started initiating various phases of 'Unlock', opening up many sectors of the economy.

The suddenness of the lockdown put migrants in perilous conditions, led to terrible scenes of distress and caught the nation's

---

[117] S. Gupta. (2020). 30% of migrants will not return to cities: Irudaya Rajan. *Times of India*. https://timesofindia.indiatimes.com/india/30-of-migrants-will-not-return-to-cities-irudaya-rajan/articleshow/76126701.cms

[118] World Bank (2020). COVID-19 Crisis Through a Migration Lens. Migration and Development Brief No. 32. Washington: World Bank.

imagination. This put pressure on the central government to act. It was in this context that the government announced a slew of schemes under the moniker 'Atmanirbhar Bharat,' or self-reliant India, worth ₹20 lakh crore on 13 May. The scheme was detailed by the finance minister in five instalments and was the second tranche focused on migrant workers and small farmers.[119] In addition, on 14 May, it was also announced that ₹1,000 crore would be distributed to the states for migrant welfare under the Prime Minister's Citizens Assistance and Relief in Emergency Situations fund. Each state would be given a minimum of 10 per cent, or ₹100 crore, with additional grants to be decided on the basis of a state's population (50 per cent weightage) and the number of coronavirus cases (40 per cent weightage). When it comes to migrant workers within Atmanirbhar Bharat, the following programmes were proposed, which we could divide into short-, medium- and long-term measures:

Short-term Measures

- Under the ambit of the PMGKY, food security was announced for 8 crore migrant workers, outside the ambit of the National Food Security Act (NFSA), 2013, or those without state ration cards, who are to be provided with 5 kg rice each and 1 kg of pulses per person (family). The Centre has allocated ₹3,500 crore and directed the states to implement it.
- In the fifth tranche of the package, it was announced that ₹40,000 crore had been additionally allocated to the MGNREGA budget in addition to its existing budget of ₹61,000 crore. The government argued that this would generate 300 crore additional person-days of work. On 26 March, the national average minimum wage was increased from ₹182 to ₹202 per day.

---

[119]S.I. Rajan. (2020). Kerala's Experience with COVID-19: What Lessons to Learn? *SocDem Asia Quarterly*, 9(2), pp. 18-22.

Medium- to Long-term Measures

- The scheme 'One Nation, One Ration Card,' which provides a universal ration card and has complete portability, is also to be implemented. It is expected to cover 67 crore beneficiaries (83 per cent) by August 2020, and 100 per cent by March 2021.
- The Pradhan Mantri Awas Yojana is to be launched for providing rental housing to migrant workers in cities, with private funding under the public–private partnership model. An amount of ₹5,000 crore was allocated in order to provide credit facilities to street vendors.

Evacuation of Internal and International Migrants

To address the plight of stranded migrants, the government intervened by starting the 'Shramik Special' trains and buses to help them move to their home towns. While this service was not initially free, the central government subsequently made the railways offer an 85 per cent subsidy and the state governments fund the remaining 15 per cent. As of 15 June, almost 4,450 Shramik trains had transported more than 60 lakh migrants. About 91 lakh migrants travelled on both trains and buses.[120]

When it came to international migrants, the first migrants were repatriated via navy vessels on 7 May 2020—mostly dependents of migrants. Over the next few months, the Indian government designated public and private carriers as well as military aircrafts and vessels to bring migrants back home through the Vande Bharat Mission. As of 10 September, the mission has

---

[120] *The Hindu*. (2020). 60 lakh migrants took 4,450 Shramik specials to reach their home States: Railways. https://www.thehindu.com/news/national/60-lakh-migrants-took-4450-shramik-specials-to-reach-their-home-states-railways/article31834747.ece

repatriated around 13.74 lakh people over six phases.[121] While this is an impressive feat, there are still scores of Indians, a good number of whom are dependents of migrants, still stuck abroad and will be coming back in the next few months.

State-specific Responses

Many states took independent initiatives to ensure the welfare of the general public, including migrants. To provide food security, the government of Telangana, on 23 March, decided to give 12 kg rice per person to 87.59 lakh food security card holders (white ration cards) at a cost of ₹1,103 crore. In addition, one person in each family would be given a one-time support of ₹1,500 to meet other expenditure on essential commodities at an estimated cost of ₹1,314 crore. On 30 March, the government decided to provide 12 kg of rice or atta and a one-time support of ₹500 to all migrant workers residing in the state. The government also decided to provide ration and ₹1,500 to migrant labourers who have families in Telangana and ration to those who stay alone.[122]

In Maharashtra, 18.78 lakh card holders identified as being the poorest of the poor, were supplied wheat, rice and coarse grains under nominal rates of ₹3, ₹2 and ₹1, respectively, under NFSA. Another 20,000 card holders, catering to 1 lakh beneficiaries, are covered under the Antyodaya Anna Yojana.[123] Similarly, the

---

[121]Press Trust of India. (2020). 13.74 lakh Indians have returned from abroad under Vande Bharat Mission: MEA. https://www.hindustantimes.com/india-news/13-74-lakh-indians-have-returned-from-abroad-under-vande-bharat-mission-mea/story-lJqr8f6jsfVfS5hgNxzzZL.html

[122]PRS Legislative Research. (2020). Telangana Government's Response to COVID 19.https://www.prsindia.org/theprsblog/telangana-government%E2%80%99s-response-covid-19

[123]PRS Legislative Research. (2020). Maharashtra Government's Response to COVID19. https://www.prsindia.org/theprsblog/maharashtra-government%E2%80%99s-response-covid-19-till-april-20-2020

Andhra Pradesh government ensured that the below poverty line families were given ₹1,000 as financial assistance. The government has started to provide door-to-door delivery of free ration, including dal, and financial assistance of ₹1,000 per family for poor families. On 24 March, the Tamil Nadu government announced the distribution of ₹1,000 to all entitled family cardholders. They were also eligible for free supply of essential commodities, such as rice, dal and sugar during the months of April and May, through the PDS.[124]

However, it was Kerala that provided the initial roadmap for an efficient preparation to counter the effects of the virus on its society.

The Case of Kerala

Kerala has had a long history of contending with both internal and international migration. Over the last two decades, Kerala has been the only state with a reliable estimate of its non-resident Keralites through the Kerala Migration Survey which was started in 1998. Kerala was the first to receive cases through the arrival of three medical students from the epicentre of Wuhan on 31 January 2020. As noted by the state health minister, due to the knowledge of Keralite students in China, Kerala was prepared for the fact that the virus would eventually reach its shores.[125] This, coupled with the fact that Kerala had battled deadly viral outbreaks in the recent past, such as the Nipah outbreak in 2018,

---

[124]PRS Legislative Research. (2020). Andhra Pradesh Government's Response to COVID 19. Retrieved from:https://www.prsindia.org/theprsblog/andhra-pradesh-government%E2%80%99s-response-covid-19-pandemic-march-2020-april-14-2020

[125]R. Mohan. (2020). Coronavirus: Kerala's investments in public health pay off. *The Straits Times*. https://www.straitstimes.com/asia/south-asia/keralas-investments-in-public health-pay-off

and had a robust and decentralized healthcare system, gave the foundation for Kerala to successfully contain the initial spread of the virus. In fact, Kerala initially garnered the world's attention for its timely and comprehensive method of controlling the virus.[126]

The reliable estimates of Malayalis living abroad also allowed the state government to plan in advance for their eventual return from their respective destinations. Initially, the Kerala CM was the only one to write to the PM in early April about the plight of the migrants abroad and the possible solutions for bringing them back.[127] It was at this time that the Gulf countries were particularly hit and a number of Indians, especially a large number of Keralites, were stranded in unsafe conditions, often without any job.[128] The government of Kerala initiated the registration process for repatriation in late April, and over 5.6 lakh people enrolled in a matter of days.[129] When it came to the welfare of internal migrants, Kerala also provided government-run shelters and community kitchens for the stranded migrants. In fact, in a response to a Supreme Court-led public interest litigation in early April, it was revealed that around half of the 6.3 lakh total

---

[126]S.I. Rajan, and Sumeeta, M. (2020). Women workers on the move. In S.I. Rajan and M. Sumeeta (Eds.), *Handbook on internal migration in India*. New Delhi: Sage.

[127]Kerala CM flags COVID-19 danger for migrant workers in UAE, seeks PM Modi's intervention. (2020, April 09). Retrieved November 03, 2020, from https://www.hindustantimes.com/india-news/kerala-cm-flags-covid-19-danger-for-migrant-workers-in-uae-seeks-pm-modi-s-intervention/story-eUgLtzaU6Yx7lsxA3qNKnI.html

[128]V.K. George. (2020). Indian labourers abroad are in dire need of help, say experts. *The Hindu*. Retrieved from: thehindu.com/news/national/coronavirus-indian-labourers-in-gcc-countries-are-in-dire-need-of-help-say-migration-experts-irudaya-rajan-and-ginu-zacharaia-oommen/article31318501.ece

[129]More than 4 lakh NRKs seek immediate return to Kerala: Thiruvananthapuram News - Times of India. (2020, April). Retrieved, from https://timesofindia.indiatimes.com/city/thiruvananthapuram/more-than-4-lakh-nrks-seek-immediate-return-to-kerala/articleshow/75533329.cms

migrants housed in government shelters were present in Kerala.[130]

Kerala had also estimated and kept ready 2.5 lakh hospital beds and quarantine facilities for returning expatriates in April.[131] This number was based on the Kerala Migration Survey estimates and the prediction that 3–5 lakh were likely to return.[132] The recent upsurge in infections across Kerala, indeed in India, is a look at how unprepared the world had been to limit the spread of the virus. However, Kerala still remains much better, limiting the number of infections and deaths when compared to most other Indian states, which, at the time of writing, clocked the highest daily cases of infections and deaths in the world. Kerala's constant engagement with migration issues through the Kerala model of migration surveys, helped to handle both the internal and international migrant crisis compared to some of the disturbing scenes and humanitarian crisis in other states in India's post-independence history.

Missed Opportunities and Immediate Policy Attention

The implementation of the lockdown showed a lack of cognisance of the migrants and their issues, both by the central and state governments. Instead of a four-hour notice, if the government had given a week's notice, with emergency transport provisions

---

[130]Kerala Govt Running 65% of Shelter Camps for Migrants After Lockdown: Centre to SC. (2020, April). Retrieved November 03, 2020, from https://thewire.in/law/kerala-centre-supreme-court-lockdown-migrant-labourers-shelter

[131]Paravath, B. (2020, April). Kerala prepares 2.5 lakh rooms to quarantine returning expats. Retrieved November 03, 2020, from https://english.mathrubhumi.com/news/kerala/kerala-prepares-2-5-lakh-rooms-to-quarantine-returning-expats-1.4689751

[132]S.I. Rajan and Sumeeta M. (2020). Women workers on the move. In S.I. Rajan and M. Sumeeta (Eds.), *Handbook on internal migration in India*. New Delhi: Sage.

for migrants to reach home, we could have avoided half the havoc. When it comes to the relief policies, the implementation of all the schemes put forward in the PMGKY requires overcoming of various logistical hurdles. For instance, the disparity in the distribution of PDS shops across India and the added demand will eventually lead to a deficit in foodgrains. Moreover, it should be noted that the 8 crore beneficiaries also translate to 8 crore families or 36 crore individuals dependent on migration. Given the average nutritional requirement of 2,400 and 2,100 calories per person per day in rural and urban areas, respectively, the enabling of food security is of utmost importance. Though the government announced a package, it will not be enough in the future. The non-portability of PDS services across state lines is one of the biggest hurdles for long-distance migrants.[133] Food security needs to be ensured through portability of the ration card through the PDS schemes to fight starvation and malnutrition. The One Nation, One Ration Card scheme will be implemented only next year, if at all.

In addition, the housing scheme, which is stated to take at least one year to be implemented, does very little to alleviate the ongoing suffering of the urban migrants. The lockdown has cut all sources of income, and not many schemes have focused on the short-term alleviation of financial stress. The package has failed to recognize the immediate distress of migrants. In light of the fact that the Indian economy is set to see a contraction in growth in the coming year[134], in order to stimulate the migration process in India, certain immediate steps need to be taken.

Steps for Inclusive Development

---

[133]R. Srivastava. (2020). *Vulnerable internal migrants in India and portability of social security and entitlements.* Delhi: Institute for Human Development.
[134]World Bank. (2020). Global Economic Prospects: Pandemic, Recession and The Global Economy in Crisis. Washington: World Bank.

Cash Transfers as Social Protection

The government missed a huge opportunity to announce at least an ex-gratia payment to every migrant worker in the form of ₹25,000 in terms of a cash transfer. This would be a compensation for the lost man-days of work and wages for migrant workers during the two-month lockdown. Cash transfers are the most efficient way to stimulate the economy, which was seen even in the case of the US, which provided a $1,200 stimulus check for three months to taxpayers as part of a $1 trillion stabilization programme.[135] Even if we were to send a sum of ₹25,000 to every inter-state and inter-district migrant worker, earlier estimated at 140 million, this would amount to a total of ₹3,50,00 crore—one-sixth of the package announced. This amount would have been far more useful in helping the workers to gain back some of the payment they lost during the lockdown and provided some form of relief to overcome their desperation, making them self-reliant in the true sense of the term.

Revival of Animal Spirits

The aforementioned amount could have also stimulated local economies by giving a sizeable number of the population the purchasing power it currently lacks. This will go a long way in the revival of 'animal spirits', as John Maynard Keynes once famously put it, within the depressed rural economies, as immediate cash transfers will kick-start a multiplier effect once economic normality resumes. On the production side, the government should ensure proper financing and credit lines among other incentives to help revive industries. This makes sure that migrants have an incentive to return to destinations that they currently will be wary of.

---

[135] E. Sullivan. (2020). 5 Takeaways From the Coronavirus Economic Relief Package. Retrieved from https://www.nytimes.com/2020/03/19/us/politics/1200-dollar-stimulus-check-coronavirus.html

Having them register for cash transfers, either at the states of origin or destination, would have given the various governments an accurate estimate of the number of stranded migrants—something that we crucially lack at present.

Expansion of the NREGA

When it comes to the NREGA, it has proven to be the most robust social security net during the crisis. Along with an increase in the allocated budget and a certain increase in person-days of work, it is also important to increase the days of work to at least 180–200 days per year, or at least 15 days per month. This may still cover only a fraction of their earnings from their work at the destinations. However, it is still a rights-based security net that also needs to be extended to urban areas.

Skilling to Re-migrate and Emigration Promotion

When it comes to international migrants, the government should ensure that existing migration corridors remain open and accessible for migrants. Not all returning migrants will be coming back under similar circumstances. While some will be returning as a normal course of the end of tenure, others will be returning after losing their livelihoods. Some of them will be returning to remigrate after the pandemic. However, the pandemic, while curtailing migration in the short run, will certainly open up new avenues for migration. It is important that Indian workers have access to these corridors, especially in the high-skilled migration corridors to the developed OECD countries in the West and East Asia, which will vie for migrant workers in the future. This can be ensured by promoting skilling upgradation programmes through the National Skill Development Council or through the states, as is done through the Non Resident Keralites Affairs, or NORKA Roots, in Kerala. This ensures that once migration commences, more Indian workers can avail better jobs abroad and have better bargaining powers at the respective destinations. This will also ensure that higher remittances are sent back to India.

However, in order to ensure this, the government will have to replace its current policy of 'emigration management' to one of 'emigration promotion', as in countries such as Sri Lanka and the Philippines. This also needs to be included in the Draft Emigration Bill of 2019, which seeks to reimagine the emigration process in India. Given the impending period of economic tightening in India, the country should make use of India's demographic dividend, which is set to end in a couple of decades. We cannot afford to waste a generation of workers in this period. It is high time that emigration promotion is pursued as an active policy in order to ensure that the coming generations have avenues for gainful employment and productivity. Similar efforts need to be taken for the rehabilitation and reintegration of return migrants, who have returned for good into the local economy and society.

Migrant workers have traditionally been at the periphery of government policymaking as they are an invisible vote bank. A large number of them cannot cast their vote in their hometowns owing to the nature of their work. This empowerment is the only way forward for even the states to ensure a sustainable progress in the post-crisis world.

◆

S. Irudaya Rajan is a professor at the Centre for Development Studies, Kerala, and chair of the World Bank's KNOMAD (short for The Global Knowledge Partnership on Migration and Development) Thematic Group on Internal Migration and Urbanization. He is the editor of the *India Migration Report and South Asia Migration Report*, published by Routledge, and *Handbook of Internal Migration in India*, published by Sage. He is also the founder editor-in-chief, *Journal of Migration and Development*, published by Taylor and Francis.

NEW ECONOMY

BOUNCING BACK: TECHNOLOGY AND SUNRISE SECTORS

Amitabh Kant

From a suspicious viral infection in China to over 2.1 crore cases and 7.8 lakh deaths across the world in the span of a few months, the COVID-19 pandemic has pressurized health systems and economies alike, including in some of the most developed countries.

To curb the spread of COVID-19, the Government of India imposed a nationwide lockdown in the last week of March 2020. The initial national lockdown was a timely and necessary intervention for preparing the health system, for making citizens conscious about health and hygiene, as well as for putting in place the necessary protocols and guidelines for adoption by states. In order to minimize economic hardships, the central government progressively eased the curbs, and the power of decision-making with respect to lockdowns was increasingly decentralized to the states. Despite being resource-constrained and densely populated, a timely lockdown and rapid augmentation of infrastructure by India have helped to keep the cases and deaths per million of population considerably lower as compared to other countries.

On the economic front, despite the challenges posed by the pandemic, India has been able to attract an FDI of over $38 billion, indicating the underlying confidence of investors in the Indian economy. While FDI fell by 1 per cent in 2019 globally, it increased by 16 per cent in India.

Green shoots in the economy are now visible. The Purchasing Managers' Index has rebounded from 27.4 in April 2020 to 47.2 in June 2020.[136] Tax collections are also picking up, as the e-Way Bill generated under the GST has returned to pre-COVID-19 levels. Rural demand is leading recovery, as sales of key agriculture inputs have revived. Tractor sales in May 2020 (approximately 65,000) were the same as in February 2020 and higher than the figure of November 2019 (approximately 60,000). Fiscal monetary measures and a reform-based stimulus package, including agriculture marketing reforms, are enabling the economy's revival.

Beyond short-term policy measures, we must continue to build on the reforms already undertaken in various areas over the last few years, as well as focus on a handful of sunrise sectors that can catalyze sustainable high growth and job creation in the country. Technology and data are key enablers and growth drivers across sectors, which will allow us to achieve the size and scale we desire.

Immediate Policy Response of the Government to Deal with COVID-19

As the COVID-19 crisis began unfolding in India, the government geared up its response with the twin goals of saving both lives and livelihoods.

To tackle the public health emergency, the PM constituted 11 Empowered Groups for planning and ensuring quick implementation of decisions taken to check the spread of COVID-19. Set up under the Disaster Management Act, each of these groups of senior officials has been responsible for overseeing and coordinating a variety of vital tasks, including

---

[136]India Nikkei Markit Manufacturing Purchasing Managers Index (PMI) - Investing.com. (n.d.). Retrieved from https://in.investing.com/economic-calendar/indian-nikkei-markit-manufacturing-pmi-754, last accessed 15 September 2020.

medical emergency management; expansion of COVID-specific health infrastructure; production and distribution of essential medical equipment such as Personal Protective Equipment (PPE), masks, gloves and ventilators; augmentation of human resources; catalyzing behaviour change as well as galvanizing the private sector and civil society to work in close partnership with the government to address the various health and economic challenges posed by the pandemic.

One path-breaking outcome of public-private partnerships during COVID times has been the launch of the Aarogya Setu mobile application for Bluetooth-based contact tracing, syndromic mapping and information dissemination. The application clocked more than 130 million registrations within 100 days of its launch, making it one of the fastest-growing mobile phone applications globally.

Successes have also been achieved in the manufacture of medical supplies and diagnostics, which play a crucial role in the fight against COVID-19. In the pre-COVID era, India produced virtually no PPE kits domestically; however, we are now able to manufacture 450,000 PPE kits per day through over 6,000 certified companies. In fact, production of PPE kits, ventilators and N-95 masks has been ramped up to the extent that India has not only become self-sufficient in this regard but can also export to other countries.

In addition to the private sector, partnerships with civil society organizations (CSOs) and NGOs have also proven to be highly beneficial. Over the last few months, around 92,000 CSOs/NGOs have been mobilized to assist district administrations across the country in identifying hotspots and deputing volunteers, delivering essential services to the vulnerable, as well as creating awareness about personal hygiene, social distancing and home isolation.

On the economic front, the PMGKY package was announced as early as March 2020. Under this scheme, ₹1.70 lakh crore was allocated for food grain distribution and DCT to the poor and vulnerable sections. The provision of benefits under the scheme was subsequently extended till November 2020. The One Nation, One Ration Card initiative was also launched for ensuring that migrant workers can avail rations across the country. By June 2020, free foodgrains had reached 80 crore beneficiaries and direct payments were made to 8.94 crore farmers.

The Government of India also decided to advance three months' pension to nearly 3 crore widows, senior citizens and persons with disabilities in the first week of April. Between April and August 2020, over 20 lakh people subscribed to the Atal Pension Yojana, bringing the total base under the government-backed pension scheme to 2.10 crore, as per data from the Pension Fund Regulatory and Development Authority.

To strengthen India's position as a preferred destination for global investors, an empowered group of secretaries to the Government of India was constituted to facilitate investment proposals with a focus on promoting synergies, enabling timely clearances as well as ensuring policy consistency and stability. Dedicated cells for development of investible projects in partnership with state governments are also to be constituted in various central ministries and departments.

With the launch of the Aatmanirbhar Bharat initiative by the PM, India can turn the COVID-19 crisis into an opportunity. Reforms are underway in a number of sectors in alignment with this vision. In agriculture, steps have been taken to provide an impetus to post-harvest activities, wholesale and retail marketing, as well as procurement operations in light of COVID-19. Significant reforms have been undertaken, including amendments to the Essential Commodities Act 1955 to incentivize private sector investment, contract farming, provisioning of concessional credit to farmers and support for the fishing community. An Agriculture Infrastructure Investment Fund worth ₹1 lakh crore has also been proposed, in addition to 100 per cent FDI in the food processing sector via the automatic route. These reforms will create multiple avenues for farmers to sell their produce and bring in investments across the cold chain.

Chart 1: Laying the Foundations of Sustained Growth— Aatmanirbhar Bharat

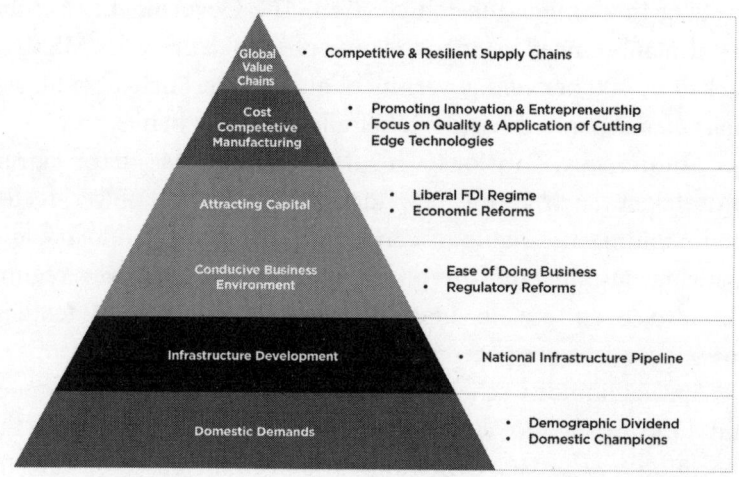

To demonopolize the coal sector and enable competition, transparency as well as private sector participation, liberalized entry norms and provisions for revenue-sharing have been introduced. Commercial coal mining, which commenced in the country from June 2020, will go a long way towards reducing India's import dependency in this sector. India imported nearly ₹2 lakh crore worth of coal during the last fiscal year. Composite exploration has also been permitted, as has 100 per cent FDI through the automatic route.

Several important steps have been taken in the defence, aviation and space sectors as well. The FDI limit in defence manufacturing under the automatic route has been raised from

49 per cent to 74 per cent. A project management unit will now be established for completing the defence procurement process in a time-bound manner. Further, the tax regime for aircraft maintenance, repair and overhaul has been liberalized, and private sector participation has been allowed in space-based services.

To give a fillip to the MSME sector, an upward revision in the definition of MSMEs has been announced to catalyze higher levels of investment and job creation. The Government of India has also announced loans to the tune of ₹3 lakh crore for MSMEs, backed by 100 per cent government guarantees. Such a credit risk guarantee scheme can aid capital allocation by banks.

Additionally, various regulatory reforms have been undertaken, such as the new tariff policy in the power sector for upholding the rights of consumers, promoting industry and ensuring sustainability. A production-linked incentives regime has also been put in place for mobile telephones, textiles, pharmaceuticals and medical devices.

Special liquidity schemes for non-banking finance companies and housing finance companies have been launched, and the allocation for the MGNREGA has also been increased by ₹40,000 crore. Moreover, borrowing limits for states have been increased, and policy support has been provided by the RBI in the form of lowering of policy rates and infusion of liquidity in markets.

Focus Areas for Realizing the 'Aatmanirbhar Bharat' Vision

A single-minded pursuit of resilience, reforms and growth is necessary. Of course, we also have to ensure that this rapid growth is inclusive, sustainable and regionally balanced. In the social sectors, our focus must be on providing high-quality school education for all children, accessible and affordable higher education as well as universal health coverage. Physical infrastructure creation must include works on roads, railways, seaports, airports, urban transport, gas and electric transmission and inland waterways. We must push for a huge expansion in electric vehicles (EVs) and in shared and connected mobility.

Economic growth should not be at loggerheads with environmental sustainability. It is crucial that we make India pollution free. The country has already taken important strides in this direction through initiatives in areas such as clean mobility, renewable energy and solid waste management. Through the Swachh Bharat Mission, we have been successful in addressing the challenge of open defecation. These efforts must continue alongside initiatives for enhancing the forest cover. We must also work towards universalization of the Digital India initiative across government and private sectors. Rural industrialization and agro-processing should be accelerated through the use of modern technologies for generating large-scale employment.

The COVID-19 crisis offers an opportunity to think afresh, undertake structural reforms and technological innovation, as well as experiment with new areas of growth. Japan, South Korea and China have all used times of crisis at different points in their history for rapid transformation and sustained high growth. All of them seized opportunities in sunrise sectors, which are new emerging areas of growth where disruption is inevitable. India too must seize the opportunity to become a key player in sunrise sectors, such as electric mobility, battery storage, AI, 5G technologies and genomics. This, of course, would require size, scale and speed of action.

Participating in Global Value Chains

The first step towards realizing the vision of a New India that is also 'aatmanirbhar' is establishing our place in GVCs. Following the global disruption of GVCs due to COVID-19, India has started emerging as an attractive option for many countries. To convert this opportunity into reality, the government is working closely with the private sector to empower them to take the global competition head on. It is critical that we foster an environment in which the private sector can thrive and drive India's socio-economic transformation.

National competitiveness is determined at both the micro- and macroeconomic levels. Macroeconomic factors include monetary and fiscal policy, human development, as well as public institutions. Microeconomic competitiveness is a function of the business environment, regional development and sophistication of company operations. India needs to enhance its competitiveness at both the macro and micro levels in order to take its rightful place in global supply chains. A passion for quality and excellence, alongside achieving cost-competitiveness through size and scale to penetrate global markets, are the mantras we need to follow for India to emerge as a leading manufacturing hub.

Developing a Competitive Manufacturing Base

It has long been said that the route to development is through industrialization. Japan, South Korea and China were able to build large manufacturing bases and transition millions of workers out of agriculture into manufacturing. India has performed well in services sectors; however, there is scope for improvement when it comes to manufacturing. While the share of agriculture in GDP has declined at a rate comparable to other countries, the PLFSs[137] indicate that nearly 43 per cent of our workforce is still engaged in agriculture. As a result, our per capita income, which

---

[137] Govt of India, *Periodic Labour Force Surveys*, Ministry of Statistics and Programme Implementation, Accessed at: http://mospi.nic.in/Periodic-Labour-Surveys

has increased substantially, remains amongst the lowest in the G20 countries. Notably, China and India's per capita incomes were roughly equal in 1990. Now, however, China's per capita income ($10,261) is roughly fives times that of India ($2,100). If India were to accelerate its transition towards becoming an upper-middle income and eventually a high-income country, a second generation of reforms, focused on industrialization, is of utmost importance. We must attract domestic and foreign investment in labour-intensive sectors.

India is aiming to achieve exports to the tune of $550 billion by 2025. To enable the creation of global champions to achieve this target, we need to benchmark cost disabilities against other manufacturing hubs, formulate a bespoke strategy for every sector based on its dynamics and adopt a proactive approach for capitalizing on changes in global geopolitics. We also need to move away from low-value, high-volume products to high-technology, high-value manufacturing goods.

There are important opportunities in the sunrise areas of growth. To make the most of these possibilities, the government has introduced several production-linked incentive schemes, including ₹40,951 crore for mobile manufacturing, ₹6,940 crore for pharmaceuticals and ₹3,420 crore for medical devices. Similar schemes are also being finalized for automobiles and automobile components, networking products, food processing, advance chemistry, cell battery storage and solar photovoltaic manufacturing. Additional reforms in land and labour laws also need to be introduced to enable size and scale in manufacturing.

Powering Growth through Investments in Infrastructure

Infrastructure will emerge as a key driver of growth. The National Infrastructure Pipeline (NIP), which envisages ₹100 lakh crore worth of investment, will enable several infrastructure projects, power businesses, create jobs, improve ease of living and boost the confidence levels of investors and financial institutions. Under this initiative, it is expected that around 21 per cent of the investment will come from the private sector. NIP's base is strong as projects worth approximately 40 per cent of the expected total investment are already at various stages of implementation, with the remaining projects at the conceptualization or development stage. Large infrastructure projects will help in kick-starting economic activity and give the required push to construction activity and employment opportunities.

Asset monetization will provide robust and stable investment opportunities to the pool of long-term, patient capital investors comprising sovereign wealth, pension and insurance funds. It is expected that $150 billion will be raised for funding NIP projects through asset monetization between fiscal years 2020 and 2025. Given India's stable domestic demand profile, these operational and risk-managed assets will generate stable, inflation-adjusted cash flows, which match the risk appetite of long-term investors. Strategic disinvestment is another avenue that needs greater focus in order to raise revenues for undertaking capital expenditures.

Urbanization

Urbanization goes hand-in-hand with industrialization, as demonstrated by the case of Shenzhen in China. Urbanization affords us the benefits of agglomeration economies with cities being centres of growth, innovation and creativity. Globally, 75 per cent of the GDP comes from urban areas. India too has been urbanizing at a fast pace; however, we must ensure that our cities are liveable by addressing the challenges of congestion and pollution. Further, our cities must grow on the back of public transportation. States must also take the lead on empowering urban local bodies through adoption of the 74th Constitutional Amendment Act in letter and spirit.

Electric Mobility and Battery Storage

The world of mobility is in the midst of its biggest disruption. Within this decade we will transition from combustion vehicles (2,000 parts) to a shared, connected and electric world (just 20 parts). The US already has over 900 cars per 1,000 people and Europe has over 800 cars per 1,000 people. In contrast, India's per capita car ownership is a mere 20 vehicles per 1,000 persons. India, therefore, has a unique opportunity to leapfrog from the legacy model of individually owned combustion vehicles, which are hardly used. We can avoid the lock-in impact of a model of mobility characterized by high costs, inefficiency and heavy pollution. India's low share of vehicles per capita can be turned into a huge advantage by designing a mobility system that ensures affordability, accessibility and efficiency.

Steeply falling lithium-ion battery pack prices have made high-mileage electric service vehicles cost-competitive. The government has supported this movement through a lower GST tax structure (5 per cent as compared to 28 per cent for combustion vehicles), given tax deduction on interest for loans and supported procurement through the Faster Adoption and Manufacturing of Hybrid and Electric Vehicles (FAME II) scheme. India has 78 per cent two-wheeler vehicles. We have recently witnesses established players, such as Bajaj and TVS, launching their electric models. We have also seen the emergence of innovative start-ups in the EV ecosystem. Two wheelers will reach price partly with conventional combustion engine vehicles even on initial cost of ownership in the next three years. India has a massive opportunity to become the lowest-cost global manufacturer of electric two-wheelers and three-wheelers.

Another area that presents an enormous economic opportunity for India is the domestic manufacturing of lithium-ion batteries. This is an EV's most expensive component as it accounts for one-third of the price. Storage batteries are critical not only for EVs but also for the spread of solar rooftops and renewable energy-led cooking in rural areas. In the recently concluded auction of the 1,200 MW solar-plus-energy tender storage, India has received bids on average tariff of ₹4.04/kWh and ₹4.30/kWh. These are the cheapest renewables-plus-storage bids in the world and demonstrate that the days of fossil fuel power are over.

A 2017 study by NITI Aayog and Rocky Mountain Institute has highlighted that India's market for EV batteries alone could be as high as $300 billion by 2030 and India could represent almost one-third of the total global demand. Even if India imports raw materials (lithium and nickel), it can capture 80 per cent of the economic opportunity by establishing manufacturing capability and supply chains for producing battery cells and packs. More than 80 per cent of India's petroleum is imported and we spend $115 billion on crude oil imports. Manufacturing of batteries to meet India's domestic as well as global demand has the potential to sharply reduce India's import of oil, improve India's trade balance and also make the country an export hub.

Technology for the Greater Good

AI is expected to be one of the most transformative opportunities for the world. Given that the economic benefits of AI will not be uniform, early adopters could capture an additional 20–25 per cent of the net economic benefits, compared to late starters. An Accenture report, 'Rewire for Growth',[138] forecasts that AI has the

---

[138] Rewire for Growth: Accelerating India's Growth with Artificial Intelligence, Accenture, December 2019. Accessed at: https://www.accenture.com/_acnmedia/PDF-68/Accenture-ReWire-For-Growth-POV-19-12-Final.pdf

potential to boost India's annual growth by 1.3 per cent points by 2035. This amounts to an addition of $957 billion or 15 per cent GVA by 2035.

India can emerge as a leader in AI given its structural advantages in the availability of data (Aadhaar, UPI, GST). The country provides the size, scale and diversity of data that can fuel the current-generation AI algorithms using deep learning. India has unique structured data due to its mobile-first usage. However, we also have numerous challenges. AI in health, education and agriculture will enable quantum jumps.

NITI Aayog's National Strategy on Artificial Intelligence aims to position India as the AI garage of the world, and presents use cases in various sectors aimed at addressing problems faced by at least 40 per cent of the world's population. As stated in the strategy document, India can become a hub for developing, testing and stabilizing AI tools, which can subsequently become leaders in the global market as well.

We now need to move from being data rich to data intelligent by making available clean, structured and annotated data, and work with the best AI researchers to find solutions to diseases such as tuberculosis and cancer, as well as enhance agricultural productivity. We also need to reorient our academic institutions, such as the Indian Institutes of Technology and Indian Institutes of Information Technology, into centres of excellence to produce data scientists and AI managers of tomorrow.

Another key area of transformation is the 5G mobile network technology, which will radically transform the world of communication, mobile technologies and data flow. 5G will connect people, control devices, objects and machines, thus ensuring faster and better communication. It is a critical enabler for Industrial Revolution 4.0, AI, blockchain and all emerging technologies.

India was substantially late in exploring 2G, 3G and 4G technologies. 5G will be another world—the user-experienced data rate will see a 10-times jump, the spectrum efficiency will be three–times higher and the latency in milliseconds 10 times better. It will also connect 10 lakh devices per km^2 as compared to a mere 1 lakh in 4G. Further, it will drive IoT technology, carrying large amounts of data, and enable a smarter and more connected world. If big data is the new oil in the digital era, then 5G is the set of pipes that will deliver it. Due to massive density across devices and connectivity in various sectors, security is a major concern. Licence conditions for 5G in India should therefore ensure that Indian companies get access to background intellectual property rights from global players on fair, reasonable, and non-discriminatory terms. We also need to create our own 5G ecosystem for rural broadband, defense, internal security and disaster relief, so that we can address our critical security concerns.

Creating World-class Applications

Even amid economic challenges and hardships in the backdrop of COVID-19, significant investments have flowed into India's IT and communications sector. The government has come out with a software product policy and an enabling ecosystem has been put in place. The time is ripe for innovators and start-ups to make India a global hub of technology products.

In July 2020, the PM launched the 'Aatmanirbhar Bharat App Innovation Challenge' to encourage the creation of world-class, made-in-India applications. India is one of the largest application publishers globally, and its developer community has the potential to make applications that can become the best in the world. NITI Aayog is also anchoring the 'India Tech Garage' initiative, which works on a public-private collaboration model. To address some of India's most pressing challenges, the development of a variety of technology products is currently underway. The solutions include a technology platform for upskilling blue- and grey-collar workers

(Unnati); an agriculture platform for price forecasting, quality certification and traceability (Krishi Neev); an integrated multi-modal platform for digitizing supply chain issues to address the logistics sector (Unit Linked Insurance Plan); a one-stop platform for higher education (Samagra Shiksha); as well as a telemedicine application to provide integrated teleconsultation, pharmacy and diagnostic services for a range of health conditions (Swasth), among others.

Health Systems for the Future

With the launch of the National Digital Health Mission (NDHM) in August 2020, India has ushered in a new era of technology-enabled healthcare delivery. Under NDHM, all Indians can get access to a unique and easy-to-remember health ID, carrying details of their health and treatment history. NDHM will also offer services such as telemedicine as part of its digital suite. The utilization of telemedicine has gone up significantly in India following the COVID-19 outbreak, with an estimated 50 million Indians having availed teleconsultations over the last few months. In addition to expanding digital health initiatives, other key reforms for India's health sector include introducing a District Residency Programme for junior doctors, linking district hospitals with medical colleges in the public-private partnership mode, strengthening health and wellness centres, and initiating short-term bridge courses for foreign graduates.

A sunrise area of growth in the life sciences and healthcare sector is genomics. We need to set in motion a virtuous cycle of private investment in genetic testing, analysis counseling and therapy. Last year, the government launched the IndiGen project, under which the full genomes of over 1,000 individuals were sequenced, and the data handed over to the individuals on a smart card. There is a good case for the IndiGen project to be upgraded into a national genome mission, to supplement the union government's investments with the energies of the private sector and the last-mile reach of state governments. A national genomics platform is necessary for zeroing in on the major risk factors faced by individuals.

Accelerating the Dispensation of Justice

The Government of India's ongoing efforts to decriminalize minor and petty offences by making them compoundable is visionary and citizen-friendly. India is at the cusp of transformative change with the greater adoption of technology in the judicial system. Tools derived from AI will help expedite case flow management, unclog processes that currently delay justice and ease various administrative aspects. The government is committed to strengthening the alternative dispute resolution system and online dispute resolution, so that the burden on our courts can be reduced and they can focus on more complex cases. A framework for the development of virtual courtrooms and centres through which court hearings can be carried out remotely, has become even more critical in a post-COVID scenario.

Conclusion

While the COVID-19 pandemic has thrown up several challenges, the fundamentals of our economy remain strong. To realize the PM's vision of an aatmanirbhar Bharat, a single-minded pursuit of reforms and growth is critical. Several path-breaking reforms have already been undertaken in a variety of economic and social sectors, and much more is in the works. Focusing on sunrise sectors of growth, such as electrical mobility, battery storage, 5G technologies, AI, blockchain technology and genomics, will allow us to leapfrog and help the country achieve a consistently high rate of growth as well as boost employment. Of course, this necessitates a strong partnership between the government and private players. The COVID-19 global crisis has provided us with tremendous opportunities. There is no better time for this innovative movement to begin.

◆

Amitabh Kant is the CEO, NITI Aayog, India. As a member of the Indian Administrative Service, he has held several senior positions in government, including as secretary, Ministry of Commerce and Industry, Government of India.

FIXING INDIA'S 3Es

Manish Sabharwal

The most relevant question for India's policymakers, entrepreneurs and investors post-COVID was asked by Jonas Salks, inventor of the Polio vaccine: 'Are we being good ancestors?' This question is important because how they balance the next quarter and next quarter-century will decide which countries, companies and individuals surmount or succumb to COVID. There is no denying the pain; we have a GST shortfall of ₹3 lakh crore, probable new bad loans of ₹3 lakh crore and huge GDP contraction. But presentism—a belief that today's circumstances are unique, permanent and unprecedented—is unhelpful in policy, and calmness is power. COVID has created a policy window for overdue reform to make India a fertile habitat for employment, education and employability.

The short term is unmodellable because we are all in the same storm but we are not all in the same boat. Modern economies are rivers, not lakes; customers pay salaries, not shareholders; and banks have powers to lend, not spend. And this will stay unmodellable until we answer three questions. Are we at the start, middle or end of the virus? This matters because life will be tentative until companies and individuals know where we are. Will companies and individuals be frugal or hedonistic after the virus, i.e., will they save for a rainy day or live for today? This matters because lower demand is fantastic for the environment but fatal for the economy (the paradox of thrift).

Finally, do we have an effective solution for professions that can't be done without social distancing until the vaccine arrives? This matters because the fastest-growing segments of India's labour markets—sales, customer service, logistics, hospitality and construction—are these professions. All policy can do in the short run is ensure that disease doesn't lead to death, unemployment doesn't lead to hunger and working capital problems don't lead to bankruptcy. But COVID's short-term pain is exactly when we should take the *longue durée*, heed historian Braudel's warning against 'fireflies and froth' and focus on structural reforms rather than the opioids of fiscal and monetary policy.

COVID accelerates three favourable windows for India: structural, global and policy. The structural window has three components:

- The world of work: The life expectancy of a Fortune 500 company has come down from 64 years to 14 over the last 50 years, employment has shifted from a lifetime contract to a taxicab relationship and capitalism without capital entails that intangible assets matter more than physical assets;
- The world of organizations: Employers staff themselves in concentric circles, their organization structures, which had become cylinders instead of pyramids, are now becoming Eiffel towers—more workforce diversity and more variabilization of fixed costs; and
- The world of education: Knowing is useless in a world where Google knows everything, employed learners in higher education will soon cross full-time learners and make the sequential 25 years of learning/earning/retirement redundant, and soft skills matter more than hard skills.

The global window has five components:

- Capital markets: A global capital glut, which has made fixed income no income, with 25 per cent of the world's bonds trading at negative or zero interest rates, means that investors will overvalue growth. Our past sins mean India is the only big country with decades of growth left.
- US policy short-termism: The Federal Reserve's exploding balance sheet, shifting the goal post on monetary policy and a $3 trillion fiscal deficit.
- China: Its credit to GDP is an unsustainable 300 per cent, many of its big companies are like animals bred in captivity who will not survive in the jungle, and domestic consumption is not sufficient to substitute for global trade.
- Digitization supercycle: The COVID-mandatory global digital literacy programmes have led to a boom in software demand.
- The economic outlook: Low oil prices are a huge macroeconomic gift.

The most important window is our policy window; change happens when the problem, solution and timing come together. A crisis like COVID has weakened resistance to the overdue reforms in financialization, formalization, urbanization, industrialization and skilling.

The implications for employers are substantial; COVID suggests that many practices with roots in the Industrial Revolution need revisiting. Vertical organizations need flattening because information and insights travel fast and without distortion in less hierarchical organizations. People-supply chains need rejigging to reflect concentric circles of permanent employees, fixed-term contracts, apprentices, third-party employees, consultants and freelancers. Fixed costs need variabilization because business outcomes are no longer guaranteed, forecasting has become difficult and resilience matters as much as performance. Organizational structures must reflect goals and strategies rather than drawing circles around employees. Pruning of the middle management must make pyramids an Eiffel Tower. Companies must monetize asymmetrically valued benefits and move to cost-to-company compensation.

The acceptance and increasing effectiveness of online learning means that the biggest costs for corporate learning—travel and stay—are no longer alibis for the lack of a vibrant learning ecosystem. Performance management systems need a higher frequency and more differentiated outcomes. Expect higher flexibility in working from home, some blunting of business travel and a spike in women's labour force participation, with a higher acceptance of online meetings and paperless workflows. But the notion that offices are dead may be premature; 90 per cent of India's labour force can't work from home because they work with their hands and legs, the cognitive elite is currently making more withdrawals than deposits in social capital and this is particularly difficult for young people. And let's not underestimate the benefits of coming together.

But COVID's most important implications are for policy; the gap between India's aspiration and potential is not a lie but a disappointment that can be bridged with radical reform. The reforms of 1991 were important but, by definition, incomplete. COVID has amplified five labour market messages: our problem is not jobs but wages, the only way to help farmers is to have less of them, cities are engines of productivity, MSMEs are horribly underfinanced, and formal enterprises pay higher and more predictable wages than informal enterprises because they have higher productivity. Making India a fertile habitat for job creation needs a cluster of structural reforms.

Compliance Reform

About half of India's employer compliance universe—1,536 acts, 69,233 compliances and 6,618 filings—relate to labour. Employers can't comply with 100 per cent of India's labour laws without violating 10 per cent of them, given the multiple and conflicting definitions of employee, employer and wages. We need a compliance commission that cuts 75 per cent of compliances and filings, formalizes a Universal Enterprise Number and digitizes all filings.

Criminalization Reform

About 20,000 of India's 69,233 employer compliance universe prescribe jail (about half of our labour laws prescribe jail). There is a couplet from the *Vishnu Sahasranam* that roughly translates to 'Why did God create fear? So he could take it away'. This excessive criminalization of civil offenses breeds corruption. But more painfully this blunts investment because a China factory refugee sees labour laws as written (not how they are interpreted, practiced or enforced by a corrupt inspector). We need to eliminate 25 per cent of current criminal penal provisions and convert 50 per cent of them to civil penal provisions.

Labour Law Reform

An effective safety net needs to give employees a choice between the Employees' Provident Fund Organization (EFPO) and the National Pension System, increasing employee choice by making employee provident fund voluntary, merging the goofy Employees' State Insurance Corporation (ESIC) with Ayushman Bharat, and shifting our ₹5 lakh-plus subsidy bill to DBT. India's social security tools need unpacking from employers and location, and to be tied to Aadhaar numbers. There are three regulatory wage distortions: gross vs. net (mandatory payroll confiscation of 45 per cent for low-wage employees far exceeds their potential savings rates), discretion in basic wage definition (inspector corruption thrives at the EPFO and the ESIC on the threat of multi-year backdating of including allowances in calculations), and national minimum wages (a single number will never capture India's diversity across geographies, sectors, industries and skills). We must reduce payroll confiscation, calculate social security only on basic wages and decentralize minimum wage setting.

Finally, Chapter V-B of the Industrial Disputes Act makes factory employment similar to a marriage without divorce. This pain of Chapter V-B is amplified by the toxic combination of the politicization of trade unions and the criminalization of politics. The only way to help farmers—45 per cent of our labour force—is to have less of them. This needs expanding non-farm formal jobs to 75 per cent of our labour force, but this remains impossible if employers face an unenforceable employment contract.

School Education Reform

There is a new world of education. Lifelong learning matters more than knowing because Google knows everything, soft skills matter more than hard skills, curiosity matters more than intelligence and Stanford psychologist Carol Dweck's growth mindsets (people who believe that capabilities are like muscles) matter more than fixed mindsets (people who believe capabilities are like shoe size or height). This needs us to fix governance and performance management in government schools; it's embarrassing that 45 per cent of our kids are in government schools. If anything should be free in a country, it should be quality education (only 4 per cent of kids in Japan and 15 per cent of kids in the US are in private schools).

Higher Education Reform

The most important change in higher education over the next two decades will be the number of employed learners crossing full-time learners. This needs regulatory changes to allow multimodal learning (online, in-office, on-the-job and on-campus) and qualification corridor (between certificates, diplomas, advanced diplomas and degree). But this needs five regulatory changes:

1. Modify Clause 22 Section 3 of the University Grants Commission (UGC) Act to recognize and legitimize degree apprentices for all accredited universities.
2. Remove clauses 4(1)(i), 4(1)(ii), 4(1) (iii) and 6 of the UGC Online Regulations 2018 that restrict licencing and prescribe a discretionary approval process, and replace them with something that authorizes all accredited universities to design, develop and deliver their own online programmes.
3. Modify clause 4(2) of the UGC Online Regulations 2018 to allow innovation, flexibility and relevance in an online curriculum, which allows universities to work closely with industries on their list of courses, and ensure the integrity of purpose.
4. Modify clause 7(3)(viii) of the UGC Online Regulations to allow rolling admissions.
5. And finally, replace clause 7(2)(vi) with clause 4(4)(iv) to allow technology-driven, on-demand and credible online assessments.

The National Education Policy, 2020, has a lot of interesting ideas that promise to revolutionize India's human capital. The details lie in execution but we finally have a road map.

Apprenticeship Reform

Mahatma Gandhi articulated a 'Nayi Taalim' (new method of teaching) in 1938 at Wardha, Maharashtra, that articulated a vision for experiential and vocational education but did not find mention in the 1948 Radhakrishnan Committee Report, 1968 Kothari Committee Report or the 1986 New Policy on Education. Increasing our current 4 lakh apprentices to 50 lakh needs four changes by four regulators (Ministry of Skill Development, the Central Apprenticeship Council, Ministry of Education, UGC):

- Apprentices rules have already introduced the definition of degree apprenticeship in 2019 by the Ministry of Skill Development and Entrepreneurship (MSDE). The rules also need to include 'University' in its definition as the entity that will execute this programme and the role it will play in such execution. The university could be made the third party in the apprenticeship contract, other than the 'Employer' and 'Apprentice', to protect the interest of the students engaged as apprentices, and this is possible under Section 8(2) of the Apprentices Act.
- The role of the university and the processes it needs to follow while running apprenticeship-embedded degree courses should flow out of the guidelines issued by the UGC from time to time, under section 22(3) of the UGC Act. The brief guidelines that have been circulated by the UGC at present surprisingly do not even mention the MSDE in it while the fact is that the MSDE is responsible for implementing apprenticeship in India. Obviously, this needs to change and redrafted with a more open mind after proper (not hurried or insincere) consultation with MSDE, industry associations, higher education institutions, sector skill councils and other stakeholders.
- The UGC regulations issued under section 26(1) read

with section 2(f) of the UGC Act need to be amended to create space for skills-oriented universities.
- While doing so, a parallel set of guidelines needs to be framed, which will be applicable to such skills-oriented universities. This may necessitate changes in the UGC Regulations for Teachers 2018, UGC Online Regulations 2018, and the Internal Quality Assurance Cell guidelines. Similarly, the UGC rules regarding the fitness of universities will need to be amended to introduce a new category of skills-oriented universities, as has been done in the case of agricultural universities, technical universities and open universities.

Financial Sector Reform

India's credit-to-GDP ratio is a poor 50 per cent; this is exactly where it was 12 years ago, equal to Bangladesh, and lower than Iran. China's 300 per cent is the wrong number but we should raise this number to 100 per cent of GDP by five interventions: increasing the number of banks, improving private sector governance, improving public sector governance, ending the discrimination against non-banks, and raising India's supervisory and regulatory capabilities. The number of banks must go up to increase competition because the number of SCBs has stayed stagnant around 95 since 1947. Recent accidents suggest that private sector governance needs to improve because the CEO is so powerful that boards and shareholders are weak.

Public sector bank governance has to improve because taxpayers have infused ₹2 lakh crore in equity over the last two years, and yet their risk-weighted assets are lower than two years ago. More painfully, they may account for 65 per cent of deposits but over the last year, have accounted for less than 35 per cent of incremental loans and deposits. The RBI is making efforts to raise its human capital and technology governance for bank regulation and supervision but needs to accelerate its game.

And finally, India's payment revolution (we have reached a billion payments a month and set a new target of a billion payments a day for UPI) would not have happened without non-banks. Traditionally, the regulatory system has been biased towards banks but broadening and deepening financial inclusion requires a level-playing field for non-banks.

Urban Reform

Cities are engines of productivity but India can't bring jobs to people and needs to take people to jobs. China has a four-day weekend in February where 250 million buy a train or plane ticket to head home. But we have nothing of this kind on Diwali, Eid, or Christmas because we have 600,000 villages (of which 200,000 have less than 200 people) and we only have 52 cities with more than a million people (China has 375). This poor urbanization has created a painful divergence between real and nominal wages, and we need 300 cities with more than a million people. But cities are policy orphans with poor governance, weak resources and difficult incentives. It is debatable whether 29 CMs matter more than one PM for job creation. Indira Gandhi said strong states lead to a weak nation but N.T. Rama Rao said that the central government is a conceptual myth. The future of India lies in its cities, but today even our job magnets suffer huge challenges. I live in Bengaluru where the average taxi travels at 8 km an hour (most people can walk that fast).

John Kingdon suggests that policy change happens when the problem, solution and timing come together to create a policy window. The global COVID-19 pandemic has offered India a policy window. Rich countries with their older populations, creaking health systems and huge public debt will struggle to grow. Europe has an unsustainable combination of 7 per cent of the world's population, 25 per cent of the world's GDP and 50 per cent of the world's social spending.

The genius of US—immigration—faces continuous and intense political challenges. India has created the world's largest democracy on the infertile soil of the world's most hierarchical society. But we didn't create the world's largest economy because the productivity of India's firms and its people has been sabotaged by the 1955 Avadi Resolution and the 1956 Second Five-Year Plan, which crushed competition, kneecapped entrepreneurs and neutered capital markets. Today our labour is handicapped without capital, and our capital is handicapped without labour.

COVID offers a policy window to change this and make our nation a fertile habitat for non-farm job creation. Japan offers an important reminder of why a risk-averse bureaucracy must be sidestepped or overruled. The former PM of Japan, Shinzo Abe's great strategy—three arrows of fiscal, monetary and structural action—is a tarnished legacy because he didn't deal with the sabotage of the structural reform arrow by vested interests whose weapon was the civil service. India can overtake Germany and France in GDP in the next few years if we set off a supercycle of formal job creation and higher human capital. This needs bold, broad and deep reforms. If not now, then when?

♦

Manish Sabharwal is the chairman and co-founder of TeamLease Services, India's largest staffing and human capital firm. In 1996, he co-founded India Life, a human resource outsourcing company that was acquired in 2002 by the New York Stock Exchange-listed Hewitt Associates. Consequently, he served briefly as CEO of Hewitt Outsourcing (Asia) based in Singapore. He is a member of the Government of India's National Skill Mission, Central Advisory Board of Education, and serves as a member of the board of the Reserve Bank of India.

COVID CRISIS: DIGITAL TECH REMEDIES

R. Jagannathan

India's economic challenges post-COVID remain much the same as before. What has changed is the speed with which new and old problems are metastasizing even as the government's capacity to deal with them—at the central, state and local body levels—remains weak as before. The central challenges facing the Indian economy can be stated simply. Without acknowledging these, the remedies will not work.

One, none of the growth engines—consumption, investment (both private and public) and exports—are firing right now. In the initial years of the Modi government, public spending on infrastructure and the implementation of the Seventh Pay Commission report held up investment and consumption aloft. But private investment and exports simply failed to revive-the former due to corporate overborrowing in the past, and the latter due to the global slowdown and India's inherently uncompetitive business environment outside software services and raw materials. COVID has made things worse on all fronts, as government revenues have also crashed even as demands on its resources grow exponentially.

Two, growth and jobs have become almost unrelated variables as the employment elasticity of the economy has crashed over the last two decades. From nearly 0.4 per cent in the late 1990s and early 2000s (the Twelfth Five Year Plan estimated it at 0.19 per cent for all sectors), it has fallen to under 0.1 per cent, according to a new estimate made by researchers at Azim Premji University in 2018.[139] This means that even if the dream stretch target of 10 per cent GDP growth is achieved, it can bring only a 1 per cent uptick in jobs.[140]

Three, lack of factor market reforms, especially labour and land (the latter was made worse by the UPA's Land Acquisition Act), and unreformed agriculture markets have encouraged a shift to the use of more capital and technology as a means to raise output. This trend is only accelerating as digitization and automation trends expand exponentially post COVID.

Four, the reforms and disruptions introduced by the Narendra Modi government—demonetization, GST, the bankruptcy code, and rapid formalization and digitization of the economy—have hurt the MSMEs the hardest, forcing them to shed jobs or remain as zombie companies on permanent life support. Some of these reforms will deliver growth in the medium to long term, but in the short term they have put speedbreakers on the road to growth. As former Chief Statistician Pronab Sen noted recently[141], the high GDP growth in 2016–17 was essentially due to the underestimation of the output collapse in the MSME sector. The old way of projecting MSME growth based on organized sector growth no longer held true after demonetization and GST. This misestimation blindsided policymakers and delayed remedial actions. This implies that any coherent policy response to the COVID-19 challenges will be a shot in the dark unless backed by better data.

Five, contrary to widely held beliefs that India abandoned the licence-permit raj in 1991, the unvarnished truth is that the

---

[139] *State of Working India 2018*, Azim Premji University.
[140] Sangita Misra and Anoop K. Suresh. (2014). *Estimating Employment Elasticity of Growth for Indian Economy*, Reserve Bank of India, Working Paper Series No. 06.
[141] Pronab Sen. (2020). *The Covid-19 Shock: Learning from the Past, Addressing the Present*. Ideas for India, New Delhi.

country's decrepit multi-tier and unreformed governance system continues to play parasite to the productive parts of the economy. Licencing may have gone, but regulatory hurdles at every level continue to hobble entrepreneurship and growth. A study by TeamLease[142], a staffing and compliance services company, shows that India's regulatory thicket comprises 1,536 acts, 69,233 compliances, and 6,618 filing and information requirements. This is a nightmare, even though not every company needs to comply with all these requirements all the time. Despite marked improvements in the overall ease of doing business (India moved up from 142 to 63 between 2015 and 2020 in the World Bank's 'Ease of Doing Business' rankings), regulatory tripwire remains a major business disabler. Most of the disablers, roughly three out of every five compliance requirements, are at the state level or below. Delhi cannot reform India from above.

Six, the rapid speed of digitization and automation in both manufacturing and services has major implications for the quality of growth and employment in the future. Banking and financial services, once major drivers of high-quality jobs for middle-skilled people, are now in shrink mode. Consider just one statistic: Paytm Payments Bank had just one branch and 58 million customers in fiscal 2019–20[143], even turning a profit of ₹29.8 crore for the year. The State Bank of India, our largest bank by far, had 449 million customers served by 22,141 branches. Consider the huge difference in overhead costs between a digital bank and a bank driven by physical spread.

---

[142]Remya Nair. (2020). 'Ease of Doing Business?' *The Print.* Accessed at: https://theprint.in/economy/ease-of-doing-business-india-still-has-1536-acts-69233-compliances-for-firms-to-follow/456867/

[143]'Paytm Payments Bank FY20 net profit up 55% at ₹29.8 crore'. (2020). *The Economic Times.* Accessed at: https://economictimes.indiatimes.com/markets/stocks/earnings/paytm-payments-bank-fy20-net-profit-up-55-at-rs-29-8-crore/articleshow/76283044.cms

The development by India of one of the most sophisticated financial architectures in the world—from the Bharat QR Code to the UPI to real-time gross settlements, national electronic funds transfer and immediate payment systems—has ensured that bank branches, ATMs, cheques, cash, and credit and debit cards can be made largely redundant through the use of mobile internet payment systems. Throughout the COVID crisis, the digital banking infrastructure has delivered in spades, with cash usage coming down in relative terms. This means banking efficiencies have grown multifold, and to that extent, job growth will crash in the financial sector as the need for physical infrastructure and people falls.

Seven, COVID-19 has set off another escalatory change in job dynamics—and a shift in demand patterns for public and private transport, and commercial and residential real estate, among other things. As 'Work From Home' has become the norm, it is a fair bet that even after the spread of COVID is contained in the coming months, most companies will see merit in keeping many employees working out of their homes, possibly at lower salaries, as there is a huge saving in office overhead and transport expenses. Gig work may accelerate, and regular, full-time jobs may shrink or become more contractual by nature. In manufacturing, the use of robots is increasing in almost all factory floors, and the share of contract labour is rising.[144] The Modi government's decision to allow fixed-term labour contracts for almost all sectors, announced in the 2017–18 and 2018–19 budgets, is now being actioned by many state governments. The future is more work for lower pay and earnings dependent on output.

Eight, the rise of platform technology giants—Google, Amazon, Apple, Facebook, Uber and India's own Reliance Jio—has

---

[144]Radhicka Kapoor and P.P. Krishnapriya. (2019). 'Explaining the Contractualization of India's Workforce', ICRIER, Working Paper 369.

changed the power structure in the corporate world. Platforms command enormous valuations (Apple hit the $2 trillion mark earlier this year) as they bring in network benefits to users at much lower costs. The new business ecosystems will thus be ruled by giant pipes (fibre and wireless connections to the home) and platforms, to which hundreds of smaller and medium businesses will be linked through user, developer, supplier or vendor relationships. These platforms now rival governments in terms of resources commanded, and governments have to learn to live with them for they bring in enormous efficiencies in the supply chain. Some countries may seek to break these monopolies, but technology monopolies are incredibly hard to control, for users tend to prefer the network benefits they bring at a much lower prices—or even for free.

The rise of platform technology companies has two implications for how workforces will grow in future. First, we will see sharp skill and income polarization, as high-skilled workers' wages zoom, and lower-skilled workers capable of attaching themselves to platforms as dependent contractors or vendors earn incomes by delivering gig services. (The Uber or Ola driver is a 'dependent contractor' of these ride-sharing technology platforms, and shares a large part of his earnings with the platform owners. Ditto for Domino's, Big Basket, Amazon or Flipkart delivery partners).[145] The real job crisis is not about a collapse of earning opportunities, but a sharp deceleration in middle-class, middle-skill jobs and a worsening of the quality of jobs available to gig workers.

This is obvious from what is observable during the COVID crisis, when the jobs that got axed were mostly salaried ones. CMIE, which conducts a four-monthly survey on unemployment, estimates that during the COVID crisis period, 21 million salaried

---

[145]*Good Work: The Taylor Review of Modern Working Practices.* (2017, July 11). https://www.gov.uk/government/publications/good-work-the-taylor-review-of-modern-working-practices

jobs were lost between April and August 2020[146], down from 86 million at the end of fiscal 2019–20 to 65 million. CMIE's definition of salaried jobs is fairly wide, including not only office and factory workers but also those on fixed monthly salaries—from domestic help to chauffeurs, gardeners, and security staff at offices and homes. The revival in jobs after the easing of the COVID-related lockdowns is most apparent in the gigs sector, not salaried ones.

Nine, the domestic contribution to the economic crisis (as opposed to global factors) owes much to the misplaced sequencing and speed of disruptive changes introduced by the Modi government. In its first two years (2014–15 and 2015–16), the country was hit by natural disruptions, including sub-par monsoons and drought. The government started fixing the fiscal by raising enormous tax revenues from petro-products, but it also focused on tax compliance by renegotiating double-tax treaties with Cyprus, Mauritius and Singapore, and announcing two highly retributive black money amnesty schemes. This was followed by demonetization and the GST in 2016 and 2017, and then the implementation of the IBC. These measures sent chills down corporate spines. Many of them faced the prospect of losing their best businesses, and found their previous illegal ways of bringing in equity through the backdoor (round-tripping, over-invoicing of exports, etc.) riskier. They thus chose to deleverage at home and restrain fresh investments. The double-balance sheet problem, where both banks and companies were focused on fixing their balance sheets rather than growing them, became a triple-balance sheet problem when NBFCs started feeling the heat after Infrastructure Leasing & Financial Services (IL&FS) defaulted on debt.

---

[146]Mahesh Vyas. (2020, September 8). 'Covid-19 impact: 21 mn salaried jobs lost in lockdown-hit slowing economy'. *Business Standard*. Accessed at: https://www.business-standard.com/article/opinion/21-million-salaried-jobs-lost-120090701477_1.html

The point to underscore is this: when you want to reduce cronyism and tax evasion, you have to sequence the reforms and give time to promoters and cronies to adjust to the new realities. The Modi government's disruptive reforms came too quickly, too soon, causing damage to corporate confidence and investment appetites.

Ten, the focus of rent-seeking behaviour shifted from private parties during the UPA era to the government itself in the NDA regime. With the courts clamping down on the 2G spectrum and coal mine allocation scams, and cancelling licences wholesale, the Modi government set unrealistically high reserve prices at auctions, which left many of the final bidders stuck with the 'winner's curse'. The lesson to learn from the UPA-era scams is not that governments must gouge private players while allotting spectrum and mines, but that rent-seeking policies are bad even when the state uses transparent means to auction them.

The question that remains is this: What do we do now that COVID has amplified all our economic challenges? Should we try and turn the clock back on the changes wrought by technology and globalization, or should we try and more forward? What is Narendra Modi's Aatmanirbhar Bharat and will it be a part of the solution or exacerbate our challenges by forcing us to think import substitution rather than global competitiveness?

In the short term, the Chinese military threat to our borders implies that we cannot continue gifting that country a massive average annual trade surplus of over $50 billion. Some forced shift away from China dependence is inevitable; this implies that we have to be more open to trade and investments from other countries as long as China remains a threat. But the only long-term answer is more openness to global trade, not more import restrictions, and dramatically reducing the costs of doing business in India, whether it is logistics or power or speedy enforcement of contracts. The only areas in which global competitiveness does not matter much are defence and space, where we anyway face export restrictions from other countries in procuring the right hardware and technology for our needs. Making ourselves competitive in the remaining industries and services means getting states and local bodies to start becoming less extractive by reducing regulatory friction.

Faster labour and land reforms will also help, as will the opening up of the national and international markets for farm produce, but these reforms—which come too little, too late—will not now deliver as much bang for the buck as they would have if implemented 20 years ago, when global trade was more open. Also, businesses that would once have used more labour or land to grow output have now found cheap capital to keep labour and land requirements lower. The lesson is simple: When reforms are not done at the right time, they will not be as effective; just food delivered long after the pangs of hunger have passed.

This does not mean factor market reforms are not needed now, just that they are worth doing anyway despite the possibility of lower paybacks. The way forward though is to leverage the new technologies coming our way to enhance job creation rather than raising productivity by substituting labour with capital.

The areas where technology will create jobs are logistics, warehousing, retailing, app-based services, finance and banking, health and education, to name just a few sectors. We can now, using technology and databases, make up for a 70-year deficit in healthcare spending by investing in telemedicine, teleconsulting, and algorithm-based diagnosis of symptoms and cures. We cannot quickly increase the number of doctors, but the supply of healthcare support services outside cities—from part-time nurses to radiologists to blood sample collectors to data analysts—should expand dramatically with the help of technology.

We cannot easily improve the quality of our primary, secondary and undergraduate education, but we can get learning institutions to rethink their mix of offline and online learning modules, especially if skill sets are to be expanded dramatically across the board. We also need to replace or augment the existing annuity-based education business models (regular fee collections over long course schedules), used by schools and universities, with hybrid and short-term learning courses for the entire population, which will need constant skilling and reskilling as jobs appear and disappear quickly in a hyper-competitive world. Income streams, especially at the post-graduate level, will become lumpy as the main earnings of teaching institutions will come not from regular students attending three-, four- or five-year courses, but from short-term ones needed by all classes of employees who need upskilling. Institutions need to leverage their infrastructure better by using them to conduct more types of courses and creating new revenue streams.

We also need financial products for the gig-work age. If you are a gig worker, buying a house cannot be financed by monthly EMIs since your incomes may be irregular; nor can your provident fund contributions be regular. Both schemes need to be made flexible, customizable and portable for individual or group needs. The days of financial products being standardized into one-cap-fits-all schemes are gone. We have to fit the scheme to the individual.

The other changes we can expect are in how individuals and corporations deal with debt; the emphasis will shift from debt to equity, and from borrowings to savings, with positive medium-term implications for our investment rates and negative ones for consumption growth in the short term. The way forward has been shown by Reliance Industries, which eliminated debt in just a matter of months by successfully attracting massive foreign equity in its Jio Platforms. It may do so again with Reliance Retail and Reliance O2C, the oil-to-petrochemicals business. Not all of Reliance's tactics are replicable, but promoters need to learn to dilute holdings in order to pump up equity and cut debts.

Many economists are suggesting large infusions of fiscal stimuli in order to boost consumption demand, but while this may be a short-term palliative, our real solutions do not lie in macroeconomic remedies, but microeconomic ones. The supply and demand shocks aggravated by the COVID crisis and faster digitization are not uniform in terms of impact across sectors. High-touch services sectors have been more impacted by the COVID-induced lockdowns and social distancing norms. This implies that demand for office spaces may be impacted, and also private and public transport. If people are less willing to borrow to buy a house, demand for rental spaces may rise. Tourism and hospitality will take a long time to recover, even as demand for digital services expand. A macro stimulus that is sector-neutral is not going to work beyond a point. Also, the need to boost jobs rather than just growth implies that sectors with high employment elasticities must be helped more than capital-intensive sectors.

The biggest changes we need are in government and bureaucracy, where things move too slowly, and fast learning is practically impossible. Our courts and legal systems are simply too dilatory to adapt to the modern-day need for speed and agility. Major reforms are needed in the police and legal systems, and not just at the level of the higher judiciary. Delivery of justice and quick enforcement of contracts will remain an impossible dream in the current structure.

At the government level, a simple solution would be to devolve power lower and lower down, so that the temptation to decide all things in Delhi or state capitals is reduced. This way, more local-level governance innovations become possible and best practices can be emulated. Skills, needs and resources are best understood at the local level.

If one were to focus on the three most important reforms post-COVID, it would be devolution, devolution and more devolution of political and economic power. Cities, states and local bodies are most likely to be business- and job-enablers when they know that they have the power to change lives and livelihoods in their own jurisdictions. Right now, that is simply not possible in our top-down system of governance.

Logically, it follows that stodgy and slow-footed governance cannot deliver the required agility in policies that enable the new economy, where threats are converted to opportunities. But this means governments must seek more partnerships with private players in order to become more responsive to challenges. This implies a greater degree of trust between business and the state, and bigger roles for bona fide NGOs in the social sector, especially health and education. Governments may grow in terms of scale of spending in the post-COVID world, but the role of the state in economic activity outside of welfare delivery, defence, internal security and the provision of public goods has to shrink. Neither state nor citizen nor businesses can expect to continue as though nothing has changed. COVID has pulled the rug from under everybody.

◆

R. Jagannathan is a senior journalist who has been the editor, *The Financial Express*, BusinessWorld, Business Today, *Forbes India*, *DNA* and Moneycontrol. He is currently the editorial director of *Swarajya* magazine.

GLOSSARY

AI	:	artificial intelligence
API	:	active pharmaceutical ingredient
ASEAN	:	Association of Southeast Asian Nations
BE	:	budget estimate
BIMSTEC	:	Bay of Bengal Initiative for Multi-Sectoral Technical and Economic Cooperation
BJP	:	Bharatiya Janata Party
BoP	:	balance of payments
BSE	:	Bombay Stock Exchange
CAD	:	current account deficit
CAGR	:	compound annual growth rate
CEPA	:	comprehensive economic partnership agreement
CM	:	Chief Minister
CMIE	:	Centre for Monitoring of Indian Economy
CPI	:	Consumer price index
CPTPP	:	Comprehensive and Progressive Agreement for Trans-Pacific Partnership
CSO	:	civil society organization
CWS	:	current weekly status
DBY	:	Direct Benefit Transfer
DCT	:	Direct cash transfer
DGCI&S	:	Directorate General of Commercial Intelligence and Statistics
DPD	:	direct port delivery
DPE	:	direct port export
DSO	:	District Surveillance Officer

DSU	:	District Surveillance Unit
EFPO	:	Employees' Provident Fund Organization
EMI	:	equated monthly instalment
EPUI	:	Economic Policy Uncertainty Index
ESIC	:	Employees' State Insurance Corporation
EU	:	European Union
EV	:	electric vehicle
EY	:	Ernst & Young
FDI	:	foreign direct investment
FPDC	:	flexible pool for communicable diseases
FRBM	:	Fiscal Responsibility and Budget Management
FTA	:	free trade agreement
GDP	:	gross domestic product
GFCE	:	government's final consumption expenditure
GFCF	:	Gross fixed capital formation
GST	:	Goods and Services Tax
GVA	:	gross value added
GVC	:	global value chain
IBC	:	Insolvency and Bankruptcy Code
IDSP	:	Integrated Disease Surveillance Programme
IIP	:	Index of Industrial Production
IL&FS	:	Infrastructure Leasing & Financial Services
ILO	:	International Labour Organization
IMF	:	International Monetary Fund
IoT	:	Internet of Things
ITA	:	Information Technology Agreement
LFPR	:	labour force participation rate
LFPR-W	:	labour force participation rate of women
MG(NREGA)	:	Mahatma Gandhi (National Rural Employment Guarantee Act)
MO	:	medical officer
MoHFW	:	Ministry of Health and Family Welfare
MP	:	Member of Parliament

MPC	:	Monetary Policy Committee
MSDE	:	Ministry of Skill Development and Entrepreneurship
MSME	:	micro, small and medium enterprise
NBFC	:	non-banking financial company
NDA	:	National Democratic Alliance
NDHM	:	National Digital Health Mission
NFSA	:	National Food Security Act
NGO	:	non-government organization
NHM	:	National Health Mission
NIP	:	National Infrastructure Pipeline
NLC	:	National Labour Commission
NPA	:	non-performing asset
NRI	:	non-resident Indian
NSSO	:	National Sample Survey Office
OECD	:	Organisation for Economic Co-operation and Development
PDS	:	public distribution system
PFCE	:	private final consumer expenditure
PHC	:	primary health centre
PLFS	:	Periodic Labour Force Survey
PM	:	Prime Minister
PMEAC	:	Prime Minister's Economic Advisory Council
PMGKY	:	Pradhan Mantri Garib Kalyan Yojana
PMJDY	:	Pradhan Mantri Jan-Dhan Yojana
PMO	:	Prime Minister's Office
PPE	:	Personal Protective Equipment
PPP	:	purchasing power parity
QE	:	Quantitative Easing
R&D	:	research and development
RBI	:	Reserve Bank of India
RCEP	:	Regional Comprehensive Economic Partnership

SCB	:	Scheduled commercial bank
SDG	:	Sustainable Development Goal
SDL	:	state development loan
SECC	:	Socio-Economic Caste Census
SEZ	:	special economic zone
SHS	:	state health society
SSO IDSP	:	State Surveillance Officer
TBT	:	technical barriers to trade
UBI	:	Universal Basic Income
UGC	:	University Grants Commission
UPA	:	United Progressive Alliance
UPI	:	Unified Payments Interface
UR%	:	unemployment rate
USMCA	:	United States–Mexico–Canada Agreement
WEO	:	World Economic Outlook
WHO	:	World Health Organization
WPR-W	:	worker population rate of women
WTO	:	World Trade Organization

ACKNOWLEDGEMENTS

I am extremely grateful to each one of my authors, all very busy people tackling many demands on their time, for responding readily to my invitation to contribute an essay to this volume. The credit for suggesting to me that there would be a readership for a collection of the kind of essays gathered here, on India's post-COVID-19 economy, and for publishing them, goes to Rupa Publications. I am grateful to the team at Rupa for their diligent editing of a diverse set of essays and for an evocative cover design.

INDEX

Aadhaar, 45, 52, 281, 291
active pharmaceutical ingredient
 (API), 213, 214, 219, 309
animal spirits, viii, 105, 106, 264
Antyodaya Anna Yojana, 259
artificial intelligence (AI), 198, 201,
 280, 281, 284, 309
Asian Financial Crisis, 235
Asian Tigers, 182
Association of Southeast Asian
 Nations (ASEAN), xii, 188, 189,
 194, 195, 200, 208, 309
Atal Pension Yojana, 272
Atmanirbhar Bharat, x, xi, 89, 91,
 197, 226, 227, 232, 238, 257
Ayushman Bharat, 45, 180, 290

balance of payments (BoP), 29, 96,
 107, 224, 236, 309
Bank for International Settlements,
 75, 76, 174
Bay of Bengal Initiative for Multi-
 Sectoral Technical and Economic
 Cooperation (BIMSTEC), 201, 309
Bharatiya Janata Party (BJP), 24,
 32, 102, 103, 137, 183, 309
Bollygarch, 231
Bombay Stock Exchange (BSE), 7,
 309

Centre for Monitoring of Indian
 Economy, 87, 309
Centre for Monitoring of Indian
 Economy (CMIE), 87, 88, 301,
 302, 309
Chaudhury–Mohanty paper, 148
China, vii, xiii, 17, 27, 36, 40, 50, 56,
 57, 59, 60, 61, 72, 73, 74, 89, 106,
 126, 142, 143, 152, 159, 162, 170,
 182, 190, 192, 198, 199, 200, 205,
 210, 211, 212, 213, 214, 215, 216,
 218, 219, 228, 232, 233, 234, 238,
 240, 244, 254, 260, 269, 275, 276,
 277, 278, 288, 290, 294, 295, 303
Choudhury–Mohanty paper, 148,
 149
civil society organization (CSO),
 271, 309
compound annual growth rate
 (CAGR), 103, 104, 132, 136, 309
Comprehensive and Progressive
 Agreement for Trans-Pacific
 Partnership (CPTPP), 194, 200,
 309
comprehensive economic
 partnership agreement, 208, 309
comprehensive economic
 partnership agreement (CEPA),
 208, 209, 210

Consumer price index (CPI), 30, 31, 85, 309
COVID-19, vii, 3, 4, 6, 8, 9, 12, 21, 25, 26, 30, 31, 38, 39, 40, 42, 43, 44, 45, 46, 48, 50, 54, 56, 62, 65, 66, 86, 93, 96, 99, 100, 111, 125, 126, 128, 129, 130, 159, 187, 204, 224, 225, 228, 239, 242, 254, 269, 270, 271, 272, 275, 282, 283, 284, 285, 295, 298, 300
crude oil, 4, 29, 68, 280
current account deficit (CAD), 29, 56, 309
current weekly status (CWS), 243, 309

Decentralised Urban Employment and Training, 230
Direct Benefit Transfer (DBY), 309
Direct cash transfer, 309
Direct cash transfer (DCT), 62, 90, 272, 309
Directorate General of Commercial Intelligence and Statistics, 207, 209, 211, 309
Directorate General of Commercial Intelligence and Statistics (DGCI&S), 212, 309
Disaster Management Act, 48, 270
Draft Emigration Bill, 266
Drèze, Jean, 230

ease of doing business, 52, 299
Ease of doing business, 91
Ease of Doing Business/Doing Business, 189, 231, 299

Economic Policy Uncertainty Index (EPUI), 97, 98, 310
EGROW Foundation, 85
electric vehicle (EV), 89, 275, 279, 280, 310
Employees' Provident Fund Organization (EPFO), 290, 291, 310
Employees' State Insurance Corporation (ESIC), 290, 291, 310
Employees' State Insurance Corporation (ESIC), 290
Essential Commodities Act, 49, 272
Ester Boserup, 245
e-Way Bill, 270
Export-Import Bank of India, 10

Farm Bills 2020, 166
fatality rate, 129, 152
Federal Reserve, 67, 70, 72, 74, 77, 78, 237, 288
Finance Act (2016), 120
Financial Stability Report, 234
Fiscal Responsibility and Budget Management (FRBM), 20, 21, 137, 310
flexible pool for communicable diseases (FPDC), 147, 154, 310
foreign direct investment (FDI), 49, 53, 65, 89, 91, 187, 188, 189, 192, 193, 201, 234, 269, 273, 310
free trade agreement (FTA), 187, 194, 200, 201, 205, 208, 209, 210, 310

Gandhi, Indira, 141, 241, 295
Globalization, 68, 203
global value chain, 310
global value chain (GVC), 188, 189, 192, 195, 196, 201, 275, 310
Gopinath, Gita, 226
government's final consumption expenditure (GFCE), 127, 128, 133, 310
Goyal, Piyush, 104
Great Depression, 94, 226
Green Revolution, 33
green shoots, 27, 34, 139
Gross fixed capital formation (GFCF), 15, 16, 125, 126, 127, 128, 132, 133, 310
GST Compensation Cess, 135, 136
GST Compensation Cess/ Comp Cess, 136, 137
GST Council, 47, 118, 136, 137, 138

Hathi Committee, 219
Hindu Rate of Growth, 26
Hong Kong, 40, 182, 198, 211, 212, 218, 234
Housing for All, 45

Index of Industrial Production (IIP), 82, 83, 84, 87, 88, 310
Indian Agricultural Research Institute, 36
Indian Census, 255
Indian Council of Agricultural Research, 36
Indian Drugs and Pharmaceuticals Limited, 219
Information Technology Agreement (ITA), 218, 310
Infrastructure Leasing & Financial Services (IL&FS), 176, 302, 310
Insolvency and Bankruptcy Code (IBC), 28, 49, 52, 114, 176, 181, 302, 310
Integrated Disease Surveillance Programme (IDSP), 144, 145, 146, 147, 148, 149, 310, 312
International Bank for Reconstruction and Development, 100
International Labour Organization (ILO), 29, 238, 310
International Monetary Fund (IMF), 3, 6, 17, 26, 39, 73, 75, 183, 226, 227, 228, 229, 237, 239, 310
Internet of Things (IoT), 201, 282, 310

James Crabtree, 231
JAM trinity, 52
Jan Dhan Yojana, 52
Japan, xii, 36, 68, 69, 74, 77, 79, 182, 184, 192, 194, 200, 208, 228, 233, 275, 276, 291, 296

Kerala, xii, 142, 143, 144, 145, 146, 150, 151, 152, 153, 247, 260, 261, 262, 265, 266
Kerala Migration Survey, 260, 262
Keynesian, 9, 105
Keynes, John Maynard, 93, 264

Knight, Frank, 93
Koppl, Roger, 105
K.V. Kamath Committee, 139

labour force participation rate (LFPR), 88, 177, 179, 243, 244, 245, 246, 247, 310
labour force participation rate of women (LFPR-W), 310
liberalization, xiii, 19, 53, 181, 183, 203, 205, 207, 208, 210, 216, 218
Liquidity Adjustment Facility, 9
lockdown, vii, viii, ix, xii, 5, 6, 8, 11, 20, 21, 25, 30, 41, 44, 45, 46, 48, 50, 54, 82, 83, 84, 85, 86, 87, 88, 93, 95, 99, 100, 101, 102, 106, 125, 126, 132, 136, 150, 151, 152, 159, 166, 171, 174, 181, 204, 224, 226, 238, 239, 240, 242, 253, 254, 256, 262, 263, 264, 269

Macaulay's Minute on Education, 35
Mahatma Gandhi National Rural Employment Guarantee Act (MGNREGA/NREGA), 44, 45, 177, 178, 179, 257, 265, 274, 310
Make in India, 28, 50, 217, 231, 232, 240
Mandar, Harsh, 224
Marshall Plan, 100
micro, small and medium enterprise (MSME), 9, 29, 274, 298, 311
migrant, xii, 8, 32, 98, 166, 173, 224, 254, 256, 257, 258, 259, 262, 264, 265, 272
Migrant, 45, 254, 266
Mineral Resource Rent Tax, 117
Ministry of Commerce, 5, 187, 201, 203, 285
Ministry of External Affairs, 187
Ministry of Finance, 22, 26, 28, 29, 30
Ministry of Skill Development and Entrepreneurship (MSDE), 293, 311
Modi, Narendra, 24, 52, 102, 140, 298, 303
MoHFW: Ministry of Health and Family Welfare (MoHFW), 142, 143, 145, 146, 151, 152, 153, 310
Monetary Policy Committee (MPC), 9, 120, 121, 311

Narasimha Rao, 33, 183
National Accounts Statistics, 15, 16, 223
National Democratic Alliance (NDA), 27, 235, 303, 311
National Development Council, 47
National Digital Health Mission (NDHM), 283, 311
National Disaster Management Act of 2005, 48
National Food Security Act (NFSA), 257, 259, 311
National Health Mission (NHM), 146, 147, 148, 149, 154, 155, 311
National Infrastructure Pipeline (NIP), 13, 14, 15, 16, 17, 21, 277, 278, 311

National Labour Commission (NLC), 49, 311
National Pension Scheme, 252
National Sample Survey Office (NSSO), 43, 245, 311
National Skill Development Council, 265
National Social Assistance Programme, 45
National Stock Exchange Volatilty Index, 86
New Education Policy 2020, 35
Nipah outbreak, 260
NITI Aayog, 66, 140, 280, 281, 282, 285
Nixon, Richard, 70
non-banking financial company, 311
non-banking financial company (NBFC), 311
Non Resident Keralites Affairs/NORKARoots, 265

One Nation, One Ration Card, 258, 263, 272
Open Defecation Free, 52
Organisation for Economic Co-operation and Development (OECD), 22, 60, 61, 265, 311

pandemic, vii, viii, ix, x, xii, xiii, xiv, 3, 6, 15, 24, 25, 26, 29, 30, 31, 40, 42, 49, 54, 62, 68, 74, 75, 81, 85, 86, 87, 88, 89, 93, 95, 96, 97, 100, 101, 102, 105, 106, 111, 125, 153, 155, 159, 173, 174, 176, 177, 179, 180, 204, 224, 225, 226, 228, 229, 230, 232, 238, 239, 240, 242, 253, 254, 265, 269, 271, 284, 295
Pension Fund Regulatory and Development Authority, 272
Periodic Labour Force Survey (PLFS), 243, 248, 249, 311
Personal Protective Equipment (PPE), 271, 311
Planning Commission, 92, 106, 124
Pradhan Mantri Awas Yojana, 258
PradhanMantriGaribKalyanYojana (PMGKY), 257, 263, 271, 311
Pradhan Mantri Gram Sadak Yojana, 235
Pradhan Mantri Jan Arogya Yojana, 45
Pradhan Mantri Jan-Dhan Yojana (PMJDY), 45
PradhanMantri Jan-DhanYojana (PMJDY), 45, 311
P.R. Brahmananda, 183
primary health centre, 144, 311
primary health centre (PHC), 144, 145, 311
Prime Minister's Citizens Assistance and Relief in Emergency Situations fund, 257
Prime Minister's Economic Advisory Council (PMEAC), viii, 23, 51, 81, 93, 189, 311
Prime Minister's Office (PMO), 201, 311
Prime Minister Suraksha Bima Yojana, 252

private final consumer expenditure (PFCE), 127, 128, 133, 167, 311
public distribution system (PDS), 230, 239, 260, 263, 311
Purchasing Managers' Index, 270
purchasing power parity (PPP), 34, 64, 65, 311

quantitative easing, 11, 17
Quantitative Easing (QE), 237, 311

recovery, vii, viii, xiii, 39, 42, 54, 65, 72, 84, 88, 95, 96, 97, 99, 100, 145, 176, 204, 225, 239, 270
Regional Comprehensive Economic Partnership (RCEP), 194, 200, 311
remittances, 5, 56, 163, 256, 266
Reserve Bank of India, 22, 23, 32, 155, 296, 311
Reserve Bank of India (RBI), 8, 9, 10, 17, 26, 31, 53, 55, 78, 85, 99, 119, 120, 122, 123, 134, 135, 136, 139, 234, 237, 274, 294, 311

Saubhagya, 45
Scheduled commercial bank (SCB), 53, 133, 138, 234, 294
Singh, Manmohan, viii
Sitharaman, Nirmala, 13, 21, 133, 136
Small Industries Development Bank of India, 10
Socio-Economic Caste Census (SECC), 45, 312
South Korea, xii, 182, 184, 190, 192, 200, 208, 275, 276
Spanish flu, 174
special economic zone (SEZ), 91, 312
state development loan (SDL), 121, 122, 312
state health society (SHS), 147, 148, 149, 312
Sustainable Development Goal (SDG), 39, 43, 44, 312
Swachh Bharat Abhiyan, 45
Swadeshi Jagaran Manch, 183

TeamLease, 50, 296, 299
technical barriers to trade, xii, 199, 312
technical barriers to trade (TBT), 199, 200, 312
Trade Receivables System, 81
Trump, Donald, vii, 73, 194

unemployment rate (UR%), 87, 88, 224, 239, 247, 312
Unified Payments Interface (UPI), 172, 281, 295, 300, 312
United Progressive Alliance (UPA), 32, 182, 217, 298, 303, 312
United States–Mexico–Canada Agreement (USMCA), 194, 200, 312
United States (US), vii, xi, xii, xiii, 17, 27, 33, 36, 40, 42, 67, 68, 69, 71, 72, 73, 74, 75, 76, 78, 89, 100, 129, 130, 159, 173, 178, 194, 198, 199, 200, 228, 236, 237, 264, 279, 288, 291, 296, 312

Universal Basic Income (UBI), 179, 237, 312
University Grants Commission (UGC), 292, 293, 294, 312
unlock, 31, 151
Unlock, 256

Vakil, C.N., 183
Vande Bharat Mission, 150, 258
Volcker, Paul, 67

Wicksell–Hayek cycle, 176
Woods, Bretton, 67, 69, 71, 74, 75
worker population rate of women (WPR-W), 243, 312

World Bank, 3, 42, 43, 52, 57, 59, 79, 146, 173, 189, 190, 202, 203, 231, 233, 266, 299
World Economic Outlook (WEO), 17, 39, 73, 75, 226, 239, 312
World Health Organization (WHO), 142, 143, 312
World Trade Organization (WTO), xii, 40, 194, 199, 206, 218, 220, 226, 312
World War II, xiv, 39, 67, 69, 72, 73, 99, 100

Xiaoping, Deng, 233